Praise for *Feed Your Brain, Lose Your Belly*

"Dr. McCleary has accomplished a heroic task—making seemingly complicated science understandable and user-friendly as it relates to enhancing not only brain health, but our general well-being as well. This groundbreaking book encompasses every aspect of lifestyle modification that can be brought to bear to create a body that is resistant to disease and achieve peak mental and physical performance. I will absolutely use this book as a key reference for many years to come."

—**David Perlmutter, MD, FACN, ABIHM, author of *Power Up Your Brain: The Neuroscience of Enlightenment* and *The Better Brain Book***

"I know and agree with Dr. David Perlmutter, who so eloquently explains why *Feed Your Brain, Lose Your Belly* will be a key reference for many years to come."

—**Bernie S. Siegel, MD, author of *Love, Medicine and Miracles***

"This power-packed book shows you how to use your mind to achieve your ideal weight and live an extraordinary life."

—**Brian Tracy, author of the audio program *21 Great Ways to Live to Be 100***

"The brain is the most important organ in our body and this book reviews some very interesting and important strategies for the preservation of this key body component."

—**Robert M. Goldman, MD, PhD, DO, FAASP, chairman of the board, A4M, world chairman, International Medical Commission, chairman, World Academy of Anti-Aging Medicine, and president emeritus, National Academy of Sports Medicine**

"*Feed Your Brain, Lose Your Belly* is a terrific book by a very, very smart brain doctor. Take a look, start feeding your brain, and soon you'll be cuter as well as smarter. Couldn't hurt."

—**Chris Crowley, coauthor of *Younger Next Year***

"Dr. McCleary, a highly respected member of the medical and research communities, has written a practical, realistic guide that is based on solid science. Readers will learn the critical components of weight loss and will find encouragement, motivation, recipes, tips for the emotional challenges of weight loss, and sound nutritional advice that will help them not only in weight management but in general health."

—**Wendy Pogozelski, PhD, professor of biochemistry, SUNY Geneseo, diabetes advocate, and nutrition researcher**

"This is a clearly written and interesting book with important information on how to maximize the health benefits of fats and carbohydrates in the diet. Its information will be important for those who want to lose weight naturally and prevent a number of age-related disorders like type 2 diabetes and Alzheimer's disease. If its recommendations, which are based on sound principles of biochemistry and physiology, are followed, the health of most people will improve significantly. The book makes an important contribution to the health–wellness field. I also think it would be helpful for individuals using the restricted ketogenic diet for brain cancer management. I am happy to endorse and recommend *Feed Your Brain, Lose Your Belly*."

—Thomas Seyfried, PhD, professor of biology, Boston College

"Weight loss from the brain's perspective—innovative, makes sense, and it works! Dr. McCleary reveals the secrets to protecting your brain, improving your general health, and losing weight in the process."

—Peggy McColl, *New York Times* bestselling author

"*Feed Your Brain, Lose Your Belly* has raised the bar for diet books. It has bundled benefits by outlining a brain-healthy way of eating that keeps you sharp while you get thin. I've talked to Dr. McCleary and he's smart—I trust his advice. You should, too!"

—Rick Frishman, bestselling author, publisher, and speaker

"It's funny, I've often told people that we eat from our brain and not from our belly and now we have Dr. McCleary to tell us why. *Feed Your Brain, Lose Your Belly* will be a breakthrough and an eye-opener for many readers. This book finally unlocks the science behind weight gain and outlines an easy-to-follow program that makes perfect sense."

—Fred Pescatore, MD, MPH, CCN, author of *The Hamptons Diet* and *Boost Your Health with Bacteria*

"I love the feed-your-brain motif. People are frantic to prevent dementia—and what your brain uses for fuel is critical for good brain function. The idea that there is a preventative intervention really helps drive behavioral change. In summary, I think *Feed Your Brain, Lose Your Belly* is awesome!"

—Dr. Mary Vernon, former president of the American Society of Bariatric Physicians

"Brilliant book by a great neurosurgeon who also happens to be an outstanding nutritionist. The unexpected connection between excess weight and brain problems is clearly elucidated, and the culprit is insulin. The answer is anything but a "low-fat" diet, and Dr. McCleary tells you why. Cutting-edge stuff, backed by great science and eminently readable."

—**Jonny Bowden, PhD, CNS, author of** *The Most Effective Ways to Live Longer* **and** *Living Low Carb*

"The thing I like best about Dr. Larry McCleary is that he completely understands the inseparable connection between brain health and metabolism. Most people go on a diet to lose weight, but what if they instead consumed foods that were good for their brain? It sounds odd, but look at what would happen—a sharper mind, never feeling hungry, lower blood pressure and cholesterol levels, and oh yeah, by the way, weight loss that can be easily maintained for many years to come. Like the title says, if you *feed your brain*, then you'll *lose your belly!*"

—**Jimmy Moore, blogger and author of** *21 Life Lessons from Livin' La Vida Low-Carb*

"*Feed Your Brain Lose, Your Belly* is a wonderful book that will help you understand why you MUST get healthy or risk your very mind. It is written in simple, easy to understand language, but the message is powerful and potentially lifesaving. I highly recommend it."

—**Daniel G. Amen, MD, CEO and medical director, Amen Clinics, Inc., author of** *Change Your Brain, Change Your Body*

Feed Your Brain, Lose Your Belly shows you how the most important relationship is the one between your own mind and body. Dr. McCleary keeps it simple and his ideas work.

—**John Gray, Ph.D., author of** *Men Are from Mars, Women Are from Venus* **and** *Venus on Fire, Mars on Ice*

"Dr. McCleary explains how the Brain-Belly connection makes your body work with your metabolism to speed up weight loss. The way he explains it just makes sense. I challenge you to go ahead and try it!"

—**T. Harv Eker, author of #1 NY Times Bestseller,** *Secrets of the Millionaire Mind*

"Move over Atkins! Finally there is a plan that will enable us to live thin without losing our minds—literally. Dr. Larry McCleary provides a solution for anyone who has ever wondered, 'How come I can't lose weight?' or 'Why can't I think clearly?' If you're looking for pain-free weight loss and a simple way to protect yourself and your family from a leading cause of Alzheimer's, grab this book now!"

—**Wendy Lipton-Dibner, MA, internationally known speaker and bestselling author of** *Shatter Your Speed Limits: Fast-Track Your Success and Get What You Truly Want in Business and in Life*

"A solid, scientific, yet readable book—written in a style the lay public can easily comprehend—that will help many to understand how our bodies work and lose weight too!"

—**Eric C. Westman, MD, MHS, associate professor of medicine, Duke University, director, Lifestyle Medicine Clinic, Duke University Medical Center, and coauthor of** *The New Atkins for a New You*

"This book is a real eye-opener! Being a brain surgeon gives Dr. McCleary a unique perspective on the brain–belly interaction. As he takes the reader through a step-by-step explanation of the critical link between food, brains, and appetite, he presents a compelling case for why our diets are the primary reason we are in the midst of an epidemic of both obesity and Alzheimer's disease. But he doesn't stop there: Dr. McCleary offers us nutritional guidance and a workable solution in his detailed menu plans and recipes. It's all in *Feed Your Brain, Lose Your Belly*—you won't need another book."

—**Joan Pagano, fitness trainer to Jacqueline Kennedy Onassis and author of** *Strength Training for Women, 8 Weeks to a Younger Body, and various exercise and fitness DVDs*

FEED YOUR
BRAIN
LOSE YOUR
BELLY

FEED YOUR
BRAIN
LOSE YOUR
BELLY

A Brain Surgeon Reveals the Weight-Loss
Secrets of the **Brain-Belly Connection**

LARRY McCLEARY, MD

GREENLEAF
BOOK GROUP PRESS

Published by Greenleaf Book Group Press
Austin, Texas, www.gbgpress.com

Distributed by Greenleaf Book Group LLC

For ordering information or special discounts for bulk purchases, please contact Greenleaf Book Group LLC at PO Box 91869, Austin, TX 78709, 512.891.6100.

First published as *Feed Your Brain, Lose Your Belly* © Teocalli LLC, Nevada, 2010

The name Vita-Loss is a trademark registered with the U.S. Patent and Trademark Office and is owned by the author.

Design and composition by Greenleaf Book Group LLC
Cover design by Greenleaf Book Group LLC

Publisher's Cataloging-In-Publication Data
McCleary, Larry.   Feed your brain, lose your belly : experience dynamic weight loss with the brain-belly connection / Larry McCleary. — 2nd ed.
    p. ; cm.
  Previous ed. published: Incline Village, Nev. : Teocalli, 2010.
  Includes bibliographical references.
  ISBN: 978-1-60832-101-8
  1. Weight loss—Physiological aspects. 2. Brain—Care and hygiene. 3. Metabolism—Regulation. 4. Lipids in human nutrition. 5. Reducing diets. I. Title.
RM222.2 .M33 2011
613.25   2010940088

Part of the Tree Neutral™ program, which offsets the number of trees consumed in the production and printing of this book by taking proactive steps, such as planting trees in direct proportion to the number of trees used: www.treeneutral.com

Printed in the United States of America on acid-free paper   TreeNeutral

11 12 13 14   10 9 8 7 6 5 4 3 2 1

Second Edition

To Heather, Luke, Mike, and Stella

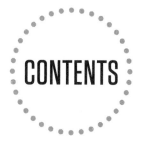

CONTENTS

Part 3: You *Can* Train Your Brain to Lose Your Belly

PREFACE

Exploring how what we eat affects our health has always been an interest of mine—especially when it involves the brain. As a pediatric neurosurgeon, I witnessed firsthand how good nutrition sped up the recovery of some very sick young brains suffering from head trauma, bleeding, and even brain tumors.

The same applies to older brains. It is well known that eating a healthy diet slows brain aging. What is not generally appreciated, however, is that memory loss, difficulty thinking, and even Alzheimer's disease are associated with "brain starvation." Scientifically speaking, this refers to an inability of the brain to properly take up and use glucose (its major fuel source). Under such circumstances, it's as if the brain is not getting enough nutrition. Because the brain can't generate the energy it needs to produce all the electrical signals it requires to function properly, it suffers the equivalent of a power outage if it doesn't get enough nutrition. These electrical "brownouts" contribute to the development of mental fatigue, difficulty concentrating, "senior moments," and, as mentioned above, they are even being scientifically linked with more ominous conditions.

Alzheimer's disease and other so-called dementing disorders have increased exponentially during the past several decades. Over the same time period, there's been an explosion in the number of cases of obesity and diabetes—even in children! In this context the question that was puzzling to me was, "How can our brains be starving while we're overfeeding our bodies?" It just didn't make sense.

It seemed to me that many of the calories we were consuming somehow bypassed our brains and ended up being stored in fat cells. I began wondering whether there might be a relationship between the rise in brain problems and our expanding waistlines and, if so, what we could do about it.

Several years passed before I was able to better understand the connection between the two. Coincidentally, at that time a young patient of mine developed diabetes shortly after her sixth birthday. As a result, she had to self-administer insulin (the hormone that controls blood sugar levels) by giving herself injections four times a day. One morning as I entered the hospital, I noticed her name on the patient board in the emergency room. She had injected too much insulin at dinner the night before and had blacked out and suffered several convulsions.

By too rapidly clearing glucose from her bloodstream, her insulin overdose produced hypoglycemia (low blood sugar). Endocrinologists (hormone doctors) have long known that insulin controls blood sugar by transporting glucose out of the blood into various other cells throughout the body, and away from brain cells. Not receiving enough glucose has the same effect on the brain as not getting enough oxygen—it stops working properly, and this can happen suddenly. This shortage literally starved my patient's brain and resulted in her seizures and loss of consciousness. That is when it dawned on me that elevated insulin levels might play a key role in both the fattening of America and the brain starvation being seen in aging brains!

As I investigated this potential connection, it became clear that there were links between memory loss and problems controlling blood glucose levels. Medical journal articles were being published that documented associations of obesity and diabetes with memory problems and even Alzheimer's disease. It appeared as if becoming overweight or developing diabetes were risk factors for the development of some common brain disorders! But how could this connection be explained?

That morning encounter in the ER provided insight into what I had been struggling with for awhile. Could insulin—a hormone that is considered to be merely a blood glucose regulator—be the key to understanding a host of brain and body diseases? That's when I realized that elevated insulin levels might explain the diversion of food calories from our brains to our bellies, much like the insulin shunted the glucose away from my young patient's brain to other cells in her body!

There was one additional piece of the puzzle that needed to be understood. How could elevated insulin levels contribute to expanding waistlines? As we shall see, there is an obvious explanation—the development of what I refer to as "sticky" fat cells. They play a pivotal role in the fattening process by storing calories in ways that prevent them from being easily accessed and, in so doing, inappropriately triggering our appetite centers. High insulin levels trick fat cells into becoming sticky.

These observations eventually helped me understand how brains and bellies are related; what role sticky fat cells play; why calories in the food we eat bypass our brains and end up making us fat in the process; and what role our daily food choices play.

Being a brain surgeon gave me a unique perspective of this brain-belly interaction and helped me connect the dots, as it were, in making sense of such seemingly unrelated findings. This knowledge culminated in the writing of *Feed Your Brain, Lose Your Belly*.

It also made me realize that just forcing ourselves to eat less is not the solution to either problem—avoiding the development of sticky fat cells is. Based on these insights, I now believe that what we eat is the primary reason we are in the midst of an epidemic of both obesity and Alzheimer's disease. The simple solution to these worldwide problems is to learn how to properly feed our brains while simultaneously starving our bellies—just the opposite of what many of us are doing.

Throughout the book you will learn that a hormone (insulin) that has allowed us to survive as a species for millions of years also has a "dark" side. This becomes evident when it is exposed to an environment that is discordant with the forces that shaped our human gene pool. That environment is the universe of foods that line our supermarket shelves today—a universe that barely existed 100 years ago.

The past century represents a mere speck in the history of

mankind, but over these decades our environment has changed much more rapidly than our gene pool has. The two are out of sync, and this conflict has created the "diseases of civilization": a constellation of disorders stemming from the obesity epidemic we are currently witnessing. These disorders include heart disease, stroke, diabetes, hypertension, dyslipidemia, and a variety of cancers.

Only when we understand the impact of this dissonance between our genes and our diet will a solution arise. The window for this to occur is closing rapidly. I hope this book provides both the perspective and the incentive to encourage you to make the appropriate lifestyle changes required to bring your life into harmony.

Because she made invaluable suggestions to help crystallize the presentation of the enclosed information, I would like to acknowledge the contributions of Christine McCleary to this book.

INTRODUCTION

This is a book about hope—hope that we will all live a long and happy life, that we will be around to help and comfort our aging parents and to enjoy our children as they grow up, and to watch them experience all the joys that we savored as children. A major obstacle to this vision is that many of us are overweight, some of us extremely so, which doctors refer to as being obese. Carrying too much weight can cause diseases that rob us of the hope of a long and happy life and make us unhappy and unhealthy in the process.

For many of us, carrying a few extra pounds has been a life-long problem. Being born large—10 pounds and 6 ounces, in her case—is not uncommon in Darcy N's family, because her mom is diabetic. (Appendix 2, "Fetal Programming," describes this cause-and-effect relationship in greater detail.) Her two older sisters started out big and stayed that way. In adulthood, they were both at least 50 pounds overweight, and, just as their mother and Darcy did, each had large babies, too. As a child, Darcy had found school to be a nightmare. Kids can be cruel, which for her was an ongoing source of agony due to her weight. When she entered college, the "freshman fifteen" turned out to be a weight gain of 30 pounds.

After graduation things only became worse. Because of her appearance, getting a job was difficult. Pregnancy was another step in the weight-gain journey that culminated with her breaking the 280-pound plateau. She was beginning to feel like she would never see her feet again. Yet Darcy seemed to eat almost nothing. She claimed that whatever she ate went directly to her thighs and "stuck like glue." Her friends agreed that if anyone was inclined to gain weight, it was poor Darcy. To make matters worse, she developed hypertension and diabetes. Her dad had died of a stroke, and it was starting to look like she would be the next in line.   ·

One of the most disturbing trends I have witnessed in recent years is the inexorable increase in diabetes. This is no surprise since gaining excessive weight is a risk factor for its development. Although diabetes affects how the body handles blood sugar, a number of other health disorders, such as kidney failure, blindness, heart attack, stroke, and amputation of a limb, can be associated with diabetes as well. What is particularly distressing now is that adult-onset Type 2 diabetes *is being seen increasingly in children!* Some children are even predisposed to develop diabetes *because of what their mother ate during the pregnancy.* These are trends we need to reverse. (See Appendix 2, "Fetal Programming," to read more about how maternal diet during pregnancy can contribute to the development of obesity, high blood pressure, and cholesterol problems in children when they become adults.)

The genes with which we must contend from birth onward can contribute to how much we weigh. However, carrying excessive weight has only really become a problem in recent times. Starvation has been a much more common problem for the past million years. What is responsible for the obesity epidemic we are currently encountering? That is also what this book is about.

But it is written from a different approach than those chosen by other experts. Our brain is what shapes each thought we have and every decision we make. However, no one has yet approached weight gain and weight loss through the eyes of the brain. As a pediatric neurosurgeon, that perspective made the most sense to me. It is from this vantage point that *Feed Your Brain, Lose Your Belly* is written.

You will learn about a simple yet elegant process that was designed to help us survive repeated famines, but which has now turned against us and makes us fat. Our metabolism has become derailed in a manner that causes us to store fat inappropriately and to overeat as a consequence! Calculated lifespan, something that has increased each year for as long as I can recall, is now predicted to decrease—in large part because of this dilemma. The brain is caught in the crosshairs of this conflict, which is why the story is best told through its eyes.

It is a story told in three parts. Part 1, "The Brain-Belly Connection," presents the metabolic underpinnings that elucidate the salient aspects of the relationships among the brain, our collection of fat cells (the "belly"), and the hormonal translators whose job it is to make sure all players in this drama are on the same page. You will learn why the "master hormone" insulin, which wears two hats because it is so talented, can enable us to live for days without food, yet becomes the culprit responsible for the current obesity epidemic when pushed outside of its comfort zone.

We are all "fatheads," because the dry weight of the brain is two-thirds fat. This fat endows the brain with the uncanny abilities it relies on to think, create, remember, and learn. It is also able to use some unique fats as a powerful source of energy. Hence, fat, which has been unfairly demonized in recent decades during which obesity rates have soared, makes up a vital component of the Feed Your Brain Lose Your Belly diet I recommend. However, fats can't be made available to the brain in an accessible fashion without the proper hormonal milieu, which depends critically upon what we eat. The foundation for understanding how to make the best food choices is presented in Part 2, "The Feed Your Brain Lose Your Belly Diet and Activity Program." This part also includes a detailed discussion of how to calculate your daily calorie requirements, a seven-day list of recipes, and three types of exercise that get you moving so you can start losing.

No successful loss of weight can occur without getting in touch with your body and successfully addressing all of the associated emotional and psychological challenges. These are presented in Part 3, "You *Can* Train Your Brain to Lose Your Belly." Also included here are some practical tips that the most successful volunteers—who referred to themselves as our "Biggest Losers" in the clinical study—relied on.

If you are not familiar with how such studies are performed, you will soon become an expert in knowing why clinical trials are necessary and will learn why most weight-loss products and dietary recommendations are never scrutinized to determine whether or not they even work. Both the Feed Your Brain Lose Your Belly diet and activity program and the weight-loss supplement Vita-Loss were studied formally, and the results were impressive. You will hear about them in Part 3.

Throughout all three parts of the book, you will be introduced to an array of helpful and important factoids called "Brain-Belly Basics" that reinforce the fundamental concepts being examined.

There are three appendixes. One explains in detail how clinical trials are conducted. The second presents a discussion about how the mother's diet during pregnancy can "program" her child to become fat. It also includes a dietary approach that is designed to help prevent such things from happening. And the third appendix provides my recommended reading list.

The hopeful sections of this book elucidate exactly what you can do to prevent the development of these health scourges both before and after birth.

This book was written for the lay public. With that in mind I attempted to simplify complicated scientific concepts as much as possible. For medical professionals and anyone interested in a more in-depth presentation of many of the scientific topics discussed in this book, a series of webinars is available at https://www.myimsonline.com/pages/Physician-Training-McCleary. This is the website for Innovative Metabolic Solutions—a group of dedicated medical professionals that provides content about diet, metabolism, and an array of health issues. The webinars qualify for Continuing Medical Education (CME) credit for doctors and other medical professionals and cost normal and customary fees for such material. People who wish to watch the webinars without obtaining CME credit may do so at a substantial discount.

Larry McCleary
Incline Village, Nevada
2011

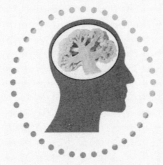

PART 1

The Brain-Belly Connection

1

"BUILT-IN PANTRIES"

In March 1963, newspapers around the world described the almost incredible story of the seven weeks deprivation of food and the survival of Ralph Flores, a forty-two-year-old pilot of San Bruno, California, and twenty-one-year-old Helen Klaben, a co-ed of Brooklyn, New York, following a plane crash on a mountainside in Northern British Columbia. The couple was rescued March 25, 1963, after forty-nine days in the wilderness in the dead of winter, over thirty days of this time without any food at all.

Miss Klaben, who was "pleasing plump" at the time of the plane crash, was happily surprised, at the ordeal's end, to learn that her weight loss totaled thirty pounds.

Flores, who was more physically active during

their enforced fast, had lost forty pounds. Physicians who examined them after the rescue found them to be in "remarkably good" condition. (Excerpted from RawFoodExplained.com, Lesson 45: Introduction to Fasting, Article #1, "Living Without Eating" by Dr. Herbert M. Shelton.)

The interesting question that arises from this observation is not how long a person can survive a fast, but what enables that individual to do so. All the hallmarks of life, such as movement, thought, heartbeat, and digestion, do not magically halt during a fast—regardless of whether it is voluntary or enforced.

The body normally must prepare itself for such an unintended happenstance. If not, all of the evolutionary prowess that resulted in humanity's preeminent stature in the animal kingdom would have been for naught. Neither human beings nor animals can survive prolonged abstinence without a readily accessible store of reserve food (our fatty tissue) to tide them over. Many observations have confirmed the fact that when an organism goes without eating, the bodily tissues are sacrificed as a source of energy in reverse order of their importance. Hence, fat is the first to go. Herein lies the importance of fat stores—our "built-in pantries."

Make no mistake, the ability to store energy when we don't know where the next meal is coming from—or if it will ever arrive—is vital for survival. Not only that; imagine what life would be like if we weren't able to store the energy from food and had to eat continuously. Sleep and many other functions would be impossible. So, whether it involves getting from breakfast to lunch or surviving a famine, the ability to store food energy and other nutrients internally and to be able to carry them around with us is a real lifesaver.

Brain-Belly Basics

Our ability to store energy when we don't know where our next meal is coming from is vital for survival.

Warm-Blooded and Smart!

An inability to store food energy in a portable fashion through built-in pantries is associated with poor long-term survival. Yet, being born human saddles us with two major obstacles that conspire to make fat storage difficult: one, being warm blooded, and two, having a big brain. A large energy demand is the price we pay for these characteristics.

While that is true, our warm-bloodedness and big brains provide us with unique benefits. It is the balancing act between these costs and benefits that we must contend with. What is good in one situation can be detrimental in another. The warm-blooded state exists at the expense of a higher and more energetically costly metabolic rate, which means we need to burn more calories our entire life. When food is scarce, this can be a real problem. The trade-off is that by maintaining a higher stable temperature, all of the chemical reactions in the body run in a more predictable and well-coordinated fashion.

Even during sleep a large brain consumes calories ten times faster than the rest of the body. This also puts us at risk during times of famine. But big brains have obvious advantages that make such a compromise worthwhile in the long run. Because of this, the brain is the first link in the brain-belly connection, the metabolic network that enables us to eat right, stay sharp, get thin, and live healthy lives.

The Brain and the Mouth

In most species roaming the planet, there is an almost fixed and close relationship between the location of the mouth and the brain. This is no coincidence. The brain is very concerned about what the mouth is doing and has a vested interest in what goes into it. By being the repository of the appetite centers, the brain controls how hungry we are and how much we eat. The mouth is the portal of entry for all of this food.

The brain must also monitor dietary contents for any toxic "foods" that might cause ill effects. This is so important for the brain that, unlike any other organ, it is surrounded by a well-developed protective membrane called the blood-brain barrier (BBB), whose job it is to prevent access to the brain cavity of any chemicals that might harm the 100 billion or so nerve cells that make up the most powerful thinking machine in nature.

There are other vital reasons why the brain-mouth relationship is so important. Unlike other bodily organs, such as muscles and the heart, which can generate the power they depend upon from a diversity of nutrient fuels, the brain doesn't have that luxury. It must rely on the burning of glucose (the "sugar" in blood) as its only source of energy.

Not only that, but the brain can't store nutrients the way the body can. If blood sugar levels ever fall too low, the brain can go for only a few seconds before it suffers from an "energy brownout," and we lose consciousness. Herein lies the significance of the connection between the brain and the mouth.

The Importance of Bellies

When we get hungry because we haven't eaten for awhile, it's really not an empty stomach but rather our brain sending the message. If no food is forthcoming, we must rely on the energy stored in our "belly," or, more appropriately, the collection of adipose tissue (fat cells) around our middle. The continual dialogue between the brain and the belly is our lifeline during periodic food shortages. It is also what gets us from meal to meal. So, whether we don't eat for a few hours or a few weeks, our belly is an important player, and it is the second link in the brain-belly connection.

Because of our bellies we have the luxury of accessing nutrients from both external and internal sources. What we eat constitutes the external energy supply. Our fat tissue represents the main repository of our internal energy stores. When one is unavailable, we rely on the other. The brain-belly connection orchestrates this interaction. It does so by regulating the hunger response and releasing energy stored in our fat cells when no food is available. We will refer to this important concept to help make sense of the dietary paradoxes that are analyzed in chapter 3.

By making proper food choices, you will soon learn how to easily tap into the large reservoir of stored fat we all carry around and how to stop food cravings. As Nicole R, one of the study volunteers who tried the Feed Your Brain Lose Your Belly diet and activity program, said, "I never felt hungry because there was no need to be hungry."

Brain-Belly Basics

When we get hungry because we haven't eaten for awhile, it's really not an empty stomach but rather our brain sending the message.

The Third Link in the Brain–Belly Connection

At one time or another we have all heard someone who has gained a few pounds lamenting the fact that it must be due to a hormonal problem. Hormones are the master conductors of many bodily functions including puberty, menopause, reproduction, and how we respond to stress, as well as a host of metabolic pathways. They are also the third link in the brain-belly connection because they facilitate brain-to-belly communication. These chemical compounds are produced by certain cells in the body and are released into the bloodstream. Once there, they float around until they come into contact with their "target" cells—cells that have receptors on their surface that enable them to "hook up" with a specific hormone. This hand-and-glove interaction is what triggers the desired changes to take place within the target cell.

Brain-Belly Basics

Hormones are the master conductors of many bodily functions including puberty, menopause, reproduction, and how we respond to stress, as well as a host of metabolic pathways.

Due to its well-known ability to speed up or slow down the rate at which we burn calories, thyroid hormone is the one that usually comes to mind when weight concerns arise. Unfortunately, it is rarely a significant factor in the "battle of the bulge." So if thyroid hormone is not usually the cause when we gain five or ten pounds, then what is the culprit? It is a different hormone. To see which one, we must first understand how the body stores fat and what allows it to build up in unwanted ways.

Fat Storage

As we have learned, fat is a storage form of energy that is portable, meaning that if we find ourselves in the middle of a food shortage, we can utilize the bodily fat we carry around with us. For the system to work properly, we must be able to store excess calories as fat *but also to access them when required.* After all, if we can't use them when we need to, what good are they? Being able to easily avail ourselves of the fat stored in our built-in pantries is a concept that has not received proper attention in the ongoing weight gain–weight loss discussion among experts. You'll now see why!

Storing the energy from food as fat is a carefully controlled process that has allowed us to survive for millions of years under inhospitable conditions. Any system that regulates the ebb and flow of fat into or out of fat storage depots must be able to sense and respond to fluctuations in our nutritional state in a flawless fashion. For example, we don't want to be in the fat-storing mode when we are starving because under such conditions we can die without food. Under these dire circumstances, we want to be able to burn our stored calories to stay alive.

Because of its importance, a remarkably simple process has evolved that makes our energy storage system fail-safe—or almost fail-safe, as we will see. However, when certain diseases derail it, we can lose weight effortlessly. On the other hand, when it gets stuck in the storage mode, we find ourselves gaining weight when we don't want to.

Fat is stored in fat cells. When they get big, we get fat. As they shrink, we lose weight. To be successful, we need to know how to control the flow of fat into and out of these temporary fat storage depots. When viewed under a microscope, a fat cell looks like a balloon filled with yellow cheese. The balloon is the cell membrane, that is, the coating that determines what is inside and outside the cell. Sitting on this cell membrane is a "switch" that can be flipped in one of two directions. When it is on, fat passes into the fat cell. When it is off, fat leaves the fat cell. Hence, a key step in losing weight is controlling this fat cell switch.

Brain-Belly Basics

Fat is stored in fat cells. When they get big, we get fat. As they shrink, we lose weight. To be successful in losing weight, we need to know how to control the flow of fat into and out of these temporary fat storage depots.

This is where hormones come into play. Hormonal messengers act like translators that relay signals between various body organs so that they are all on the same page when called upon to respond. One bit of metabolic magic they perform is to help determine whether we are in a fat-storing or a fat-burning mode. As the third link in the brain-belly connection, hormones coordinate this delicate balance in conjunction with the brain and fat tissue.

The "master" hormone in this setting is called insulin. You have probably already heard about insulin; it is responsible for regulating blood sugar levels. In addition, it plays a key role in turning this fat-storing switch on and off. Read on to learn more about how insulin regulates fat storage and why we gain weight if we make the wrong food choices. Insulin is so important in this process that the entire next chapter is devoted to comprehending all that it does.

Food Addicts!

It makes sense that fat-storing machinery has become ingrained in our body chemistry, brain, and genetic makeup because of the vital role it plays. However, consider for a moment that the hunger and reward centers in the brain are close to each other and communicate freely. One implication of this proximity is that certain foods may interact with both simultaneously.

The reward system plays a key role in the addictive nature of drugs by reinforcing their use. The "high" that accompanies a heroin rush is both intensely pleasurable and of brief duration. For continued stimulation, another "fix" is required. As a result, the brain actually rewires itself to be on the lookout for whatever produced the initial high. Alterations in nerve cells and how they are connected actually develop to facilitate the response—even to the point where it occurs subconsciously.

The same reaction can be fostered when we eat. Comfort foods are the prime offenders. They have potentially addictive properties because they make us feel good. Consequently, we look forward to the next sweet, savory bite. A pleasure response is generated and is repeatedly reinforced. Food manufacturers understand this addiction all too well: the universe of such food products on the market today bears witness to that fact.

Sweetener	Relative Sweetener Rating
Glucose	0.8
Table Sugar	1.0
HFCS	1.2
Fructose	1.4
Aspartame	180
Acesulfame	200
Sweet'N Low	300
Splenda	600

Table 1.1

Food additives and sweeteners are able to augment the addictive properties of food. As an example, on the relative sweetness rating scale, glucose (the primary "sugar" in blood) weighs in at a measly 0.8. Compare that with table sugar (sucrose) that is rated 1.0. High-fructose corn syrup (HFCS) is 1.2. And fructose is 1.4—almost twice as sweet as glucose. Where do artificial sweeteners fall on this same scale? Aspartame is listed at 180, acesulfame at 200, and saccharin (Sweet'N Low) at 300, while sucralose (Splenda) weighs in at 600. This means Splenda is 750 times as sweet as glucose! No wonder so many of us are addicted to foods containing these supersweet additives, many of which already contain loads of sugar or HFCS.

The sweet taste such products deliver can change the way we perceive food, think about food, and crave food, and they can even enhance our appetite and influence insulin secretion. Each of these factors can contribute to an overeating response, which is obviously not something those of us who wish to be thin can afford. In my opinion, sweeteners should be avoided, if possible, for your safety and your waistline.

The pivotal role insulin plays in appetite control and weight regulation, how it interacts with fat and sugar (and other foods that are broken down into sugar), and how it can easily be controlled are topics that will whet your appetite in chapter 2.

INSULIN—THE MASTER HORMONE

The ability to store fat has allowed the human race to survive for millions of years. No system is infallible, however, and when things go awry, weight gain is one potential outcome. What we need to understand is that to be beneficial, *the handling of fat must be a two-way street.* Fat must be able to enter fat cells when storage is appropriate and to exit fat cells when we need ready energy.

Brain-Belly Basics

The handling of fat must be a two-way street. Fat must be able to enter fat cells when storage is appropriate and to exit fat cells when we need ready energy.

Hormones, specifically the hormone insulin, are regulators of this delicate balance. In conjunction with the brain and our fat cells, they constitute the primary components of the brain-belly connection. As such, they control the flow of information about what we have eaten, what our energy requirements are, the status of our fat stores, and the level of our hunger.

Immediately after we eat, abundant energy is available for the brain and the body. As the hours go by, we use up the energy from the food we have eaten and must be able to tap into our fat stores. For this to happen in a seamless fashion, fat must be released from fat cells when it is needed. Under these circumstances, we don't get hungry, because we rely on our internal source of calories—stored fat—as our energy source. The hormone insulin coordinates this process.

It helps to think of insulin as the fulcrum on which the fat-storing/fat-burning platform pivots. When insulin levels are elevated, the system shifts to fat storage. As insulin levels fall back to normal, fat can leave fat cells and be used as fuel throughout the body.

What happens between meals after we have burned all the food calories we ate during our last meal (our external source of energy) if insulin levels remain elevated? High insulin generates a signal that keeps fat packed in fat cells and prevents it from being released for the body to use. Under these conditions, our internal energy stores are not readily accessible, which causes our brain to respond by stimulating the appetite centers that send out hunger signals. So, as a result of being unable to access stored fat, we end up eating more instead. This explains why losing weight is so difficult. It is because the food we eat puts us in a persistent fat-storing mode, which results in overeating. We will discuss what foods to eat and which ones to avoid later in this chapter.

In order to visualize what is happening between meals when high insulin levels prevent fat from being released, think of it as if the body is not even aware that those fat cells exist. The inaccessible fat tissue thus becomes essentially invisible to the body. Without an internal source of energy to use, we head back to the refrigerator for more food.

As you can see, persistently elevated insulin levels prevent us from using our stored fat and make us hungry. We then eat more instead of doing what we want to do, which is burn stored fat. This is the worst position to be in for losing weight. In fact, it is the optimal scenario for gaining weight. Hence, the real villain here is insulin—specifically, elevated insulin levels!

Brain-Belly Basics

Persistently elevated insulin levels prevent us from using our stored fat and make us hungry.

"Sticky" Fat Cells

The amount of fat in your fat cells is determined not just by how much fat enters them but also by how much fat leaves them. When the amount entering and the amount leaving over a period of time are equal, fat cells don't enlarge. They properly perform their job of storing fat temporarily as you eat and releasing it between meals so that you don't feel hungry before your next meal. You can see that when they're used in this fashion, fat cells are not intrinsically evil. In fact, they serve a very useful purpose: they allow you to do important tasks such as go to work, pick up the kids, or relax instead of having to eat constantly to maintain your energy level.

However, if poor food choices are made, problems arise because healthy fat cells become what I call "sticky"—meaning they accumulate calories when you eat, but they don't release them between meals. As a result, fat cells keep enlarging and you gain weight. How does this happen?

Fat cells don't make any decisions independently. They must be told when their stored fat energy is required. Hormones monitor this situation carefully, and when more energy is needed, insulin is the messenger that communicates with each fat cell about what action is necessary. When insulin levels are high, they tell fat cells to keep fat locked up and not to release it. When insulin levels fall, the opposite happens: they send a message to each fat cell to start releasing fat for use by the body. So, sticky fat cells develop when insulin levels are too high.

The Operator of Your Fat Cells' On-Off Switch

As in many other biological processes, a cellular "switch" is involved when fat is stored. Insulin actually flips the switch. This is how it disseminates its message to each of the fat cells throughout the body. When your insulin level is high, fat cells are locked in the fat-storing mode. In this situation, they are unable to release their stored fat. When your insulin level is low, the switch is turned off, and fat can be released for use by the body.

What happens if your insulin level stays high most of the day? Your fat cells have no choice but to respond by staying locked in storage mode, and they keep getting larger and larger. Not only that, but because the energy in that stored fat is not available to be properly used, nutrient levels fall, and your brain's appetite centers tell you it's time to eat again.

Thus, high insulin levels are a potent signal that keeps the fat storage switch in the "on" position—occasionally *even when the body is starving for energy.* As we will see, this happens because insulin has a one-track mind. And although this trait has stood it in good stead for many years, when insulin receives mixed dietary messages, such as those generated from current foods, problems arise, as we will soon discover.

Brain-Belly Basics

High insulin levels are a potent signal that keeps the fat storage switch in the "on" position—occasionally even when the body is starving for energy.

A Multitasking Hormone

One of the other tasks insulin performs is the regulation of blood sugar. As more glucose enters the blood, more insulin is required to control it. Since most foods that contain carbohydrates are broken down into glucose, the amount you eat determines your blood glucose level, which, in turn, is responsible for telling the body how much insulin to release. However, a problem arises especially after the consumption of large amounts of refined carbohydrates because of the excessively high insulin level that is required to process the onslaught of glucose.

This occurs because, in addition to being the hormone that controls blood sugar levels, insulin is also the fat storage hormone. The ability to wear both metabolic hats streamlines the hormonal system, but at the same time ties the glucose-regulating and fat-storing systems together because they are both controlled by insulin. When glucose levels rise, fat storage increases because of the associated rise in insulin.

Hence, when insulin has to transport a lot of glucose out of the blood, it has no choice but to store a lot of fat at the same time. This way of doing business makes the body more efficient. But when modern diets deliver large glucose loads, excessive fat storage is an unwanted by-product. And this is often what happens repeatedly throughout the day.

As we have seen, the primary source of glucose in the bloodstream is the carbohydrate content in the diet. Essentially none of it comes from the fat and protein we eat. This demonstrates how our food choices directly determine our glucose level and, subsequently, our insulin level. The more carbohydrates you eat, the higher your insulin climbs to control blood glucose. At the same time, it will store a lot of fat. This is not good if you want to stay thin or to lose weight.

"Good" Carbs, "Bad" Carbs

Carbohydrates are the primary source of glucose in your bloodstream, but not all carbs are created equal. Those that are *rapidly digested*—the "bad" carbs—are the worst offenders. Those that are *very slowly digested* over many hours—the "good" carbs—act as slow-release forms of glucose and are the best suppliers.

You may have heard that "complex" carbs are the healthy ones. This is not always the case. Consider, for example, bread or potatoes. They contain complex carbs in a form that is rapidly digested and absorbed, thus causing a rapid rise in blood sugar levels. For this reason, I place them in the bad carbs category. Most good carbs are combined with fiber. The body very slowly absorbs this form of complex carbohydrate because the fiber it is bound to acts like glue that slows down the release of the attached sugar into the bloodstream. Fiber is usually removed when foods are processed. So, the take-home message is not to reach too fast for labels that advertise complex carbs.

Brain-Belly Basics

Carbohydrates that are rapidly digested—the "bad" carbs—are the worst offenders. Those that are very slowly digested over many hours—the "good" carbs—act as slow-release forms of glucose and are the best suppliers.

Your food choices directly control how badly your body wants to hang onto fat—and subsequently, how likely you are to gain weight. The more carbohydrates you eat, especially those without fiber, the higher your insulin will go—and high is not good if you want to lead a thin lifestyle. If you feel that fat just seems to stick to your body like glue, this is the reason why.

The Fat-Storing Trigger That Farmers Depend On

Animals are not usually fed a wide variety of foods. However, significant changes occur when they go from being grass-fed to corn-fed. Take a look at how this nutritional alteration makes a big difference to the bottom line in the cattle business.

What has traditionally been the signal the body responds to when it is time to store calories as fat? Farmers know the answer to this question all too well. Just look at what they do in feedlots. They crowd animals together so they can't move around and expend energy (that is, exercise). And, most importantly, they feed these animals corn. As corn is digested, it is converted into sugar, which is a potent signal for the release of insulin. As a result of eating corn all day, the animals' insulin levels remain elevated, which keeps them in a fat-storing mode. They gain weight rapidly—just what the farmers want, because they get paid by the pound. All the marbling in corn-fed beef is just this fat being stored in the meat.

This is a very effective method for making cattle bigger (actually fatter), because it increases fat storage (meaning fat going into fat cells) while simultaneously keeping the fat already in fat cells from being released. Our bodies work the same way. So, by eating corn and other similar foods that raise insulin levels, we get fat as well. Just think of it as the human version of "the feedlot syndrome."

Modern Fat Storage Signals—Better Than Anything Mother Nature Ever Devised

When cows eat corn all day, they get fat. Corn is their bad carb. Humans don't continuously eat corn, but they work hard to choose an array of foods that produce the same results. By eating a diet that contains a number of selections from the bad carbs category, we effectively produce the identical hormonal profile seen in cows in a feedlot, with similar results: fat humans.

Non-starchy fruits and vegetables contain valuable nutrients and release their sugar slowly. They are important parts of any healthy diet. Foods in the good carb category include berries, avocadoes, cherries, green leafy vegetables, peppers, onions, tomatoes, carrots, asparagus, celery, spinach, kale, chard, artichokes, cauliflower, broccoli, Brussels sprouts, green beans, and their neighbors in the produce aisle.

As we have cultivated and interbred various strains of foods, their sugar content has increased. One example is the luscious apples we find today in the produce section of the supermarket. Apples that existed several hundred years ago were small and fibrous. They didn't taste very good because they didn't have the abundance of white sugar-filled fruit that we now enjoy. They contained less "fruit" and more fiber. What fruit sugar they did contain was released slowly, so it had very little impact on blood glucose (and subsequently, insulin).

Apples are obviously not the cause of the modern obesity trend. Nor is the fat in our diet. It is primarily the manufactured fat-storage triggers that are to blame—the "bad" carbs listed previously—combined with an ancient, evolutionarily based fat-storage scheme that is being repeatedly triggered throughout the day that has created the current obesity epidemic. It has also created an epidemic of brain starvation that will be discussed in Chapter 5.

Jay Cutler's Secret

The following anecdote will give you an important perspective about the impact of insulin on body weight.

In 2007 Jay Cutler was the quarterback for the Denver Broncos. It is no secret that you have to be big and strong to survive in professional sports. However, during the course of that season, he lost almost thirty-five pounds. This occurred despite training with weights, regularly eating thousands of calories per day, and taking numerous nutritional supplements.

How could this happen? The short answer is that although he was twenty-four, he developed a childhood disease—diabetes mellitus (Type 1 diabetes)—a condition in which an inflammatory process destroyed the cells in his pancreas, the organ that makes insulin. Without any insulin to store energy, he lost almost 15 percent of his body mass *even though he was doing everything he could to gain weight*. This observation will help you understand how to lose weight easily. He subsequently easily regained his lost weight when he was placed on insulin injections.

A diet that produces a high insulin signal directs the body to store fat, and a diet that minimizes the food storage signal (by keeping insulin levels low) usually produces weight loss. Juvenile diabetes is merely an extreme example of this phenomenon. People who develop juvenile diabetes usually lose weight—a lot of weight. This is so consistent a response that it is one of the first symptoms doctors look for when they see a child who might be developing juvenile diabetes.

Now, using what we have just learned, we will be able to make sense of some challenging dietary paradoxes in chapter 3 that will lead us to a thinner lifestyle.

3

THE CLAMOR OF HUNGER— LESSONS FROM FIVE DIETS

You learned in chapter 2 that eating food that raises your insulin level quickly, and keeps it elevated, prevents your body from getting rid of fat. Most likely you've also frequently heard that we eat too much and don't exercise enough. So you'll be very interested to hear that similar factors help determine when you get hungry—and how hungry you feel.

It seems logical to assume that if you don't eat enough food you'll get the munchies, and if you eat too much you won't. However, numerous studies have shown that this assumption is not always true—or at least that the correlation between how much you eat and how hungry you feel is not as direct as it might seem. Most of us have had similar personal experiences, so this should come as no surprise. Studying the way our bodies react to how much we eat—and what we eat—can help us to understand the *right* way to eat so we don't feel hungry all the time. After all, nobody will stick to any diet that prevents them from eating when they feel hungry.

Let's examine five different "diets"—some producing seemingly paradoxical results—and see what they teach us.

1. Calorie-Restricted Low-Fat Diet

In 1944, Ancel Keys performed a dietary experiment on men who were restricted to 1,570 calories per day—about one-half of what had been required for them to maintain their weight previously. The diet consisted primarily of "whole-wheat bread, potatoes, cereals, and considerable amounts of turnips and cabbage." The composition was 57.3 percent carbohydrate (about 900 calories), 17.2 percent fat (about 270 calories), and 25.4 percent protein (about 400 calories)—a macronutrient breakdown that resembles diets that many people follow today. One of Keys's goals was to document the psychological response to severe (about 50 percent) caloric restriction on a low-fat diet.

Result: the participants lost about a pound a week but complained of unremitting and ravenous hunger. Food became a preoccupation. Plates and silverware were licked clean. The mere act of waiting in line to be served was frequently overwhelming, and neuroses and psychoses were not uncommon. Subjects also complained of always feeling cold.

While this diet may appear excessively severe, its calorie restriction is within the realm of what are considered conventional reducing diets today, with similar results—persistent hunger!

2. Calorie-Restricted Higher-Fat Diet

In 1936, Per Hanssen published a report suggesting that in addition to caloric content, nutrient content might be vital in determining how the body responds to dietary changes. He treated twenty-one obese subjects with an 1,850-calorie diet. The composition was approximately 25 percent carbohydrate (about 470 calories), 60 percent fat (about 1,100 calories), and 15 percent protein (about 280 calories). It is interesting to note that the subjects on Hanssen's diet, which contained four times the fat content of Keys's diet, never felt hungry.

Result: Hanssen's subjects stayed on the diet from one to four months, lost an average of two pounds per week, and never felt hungry even while eating approximately the same number of calories as were consumed on the Keys diet.

> ### Brain-Belly Basics
> It is interesting to note that the subjects on Hanssen's diet, which contained four times the fat content of Keys's diet, never felt hungry.

3. Total Starvation Diet

On a total starvation diet (such as the episode described at the beginning of chapter 1), subjects drink water but eat no food at all. On this type of diet, all of the calories burned are those that are released from body stores. After a few days of not eating, approximately 70 percent of the calories burned are from fat cells, and the remaining 30 percent are from muscle breakdown and glucose. Under these circumstances, if the carbohydrate contribution (glucose) is about 20 percent, the fat-to-carb calorie ratio in the nutrients being utilized is 3.5:1 (70:20).

Result: after a few days of starvation, subjects' hunger abates, food cravings disappear, and weight is lost!

4. Cruise Ship Diet

If you've ever taken a cruise, you've undoubtedly been stunned by the amount of food you eat—a sumptuous breakfast, large lunch, pizza at 3 PM, frequent snacks, dessert extravaganzas, and midnight feeds—often with your only physical activity consisting of lounging around the pool while sipping island punch. A "typical" cruise ship diet might include roughly 4,500 calories. It contains about 50 percent carbohydrate (2,250 calories), 30 percent fat (1,350 calories), and 20 percent protein (900 calories).

Result: in such situations, most people find themselves getting hungry despite the large number of calories they're taking in, and, not surprisingly, gaining weight.

5. Typical American Diet

It may amuse you to learn that the approximate dietary composition of a "typical" American diet—carbohydrate 55 percent (1,375 calories), fat 30 percent (750 calories), protein 15 percent (375 calories)—is not too different from the first diet we looked at—the low-fat diet—but with more calories and often containing lots of rapidly digested carbohydrates and very few healthy fats, proteins, or fiber.

Result: the average American on this "typical" diet is likely to be overweight.

Let's Compare

This table summarizes some information about the diets just described.

Name of Diet	Calories	Carbohy-drate	Fat	Protein	Fat:Carb Ratio	Result
Keys Low-Fat Diet	1,570 (Low calorie diet)	57.3% (900 calories)	17.2% (270 calories)	25.4% (400 calories)	0.3:1	Weight loss; constant hunger; feeling cold
Hanssen Higher-Fat Diet	1,850 (Low calorie diet)	25% (470 calories)	60% (1,100 calories)	15% (280 calories)	2.4:1	Weight loss; no hunger
Total Starvation Diet	0 (No calorie diet)	20% (from internal stores)	70% (from internal stores)	10% (from internal stores)	3.5:1	Weight loss; no hunger
Cruise Ship Diet	4,500 (High calorie diet)	50% (2,250 calories)	30% (1,350 calories)	20% (900 calories)	0.6:1	Weight gain; frequent hunger
Typical American Diet	2,500 ("Typical" diet)	55% (1,375 calories)	30% (750 calories)	15% (375 calories)	0.55:1	Weight gain; frequent hunger

Table 3.1

Some Important Concepts

Before you learn how these very different diets can produce the seemingly paradoxical results they do, it's helpful to be aware of the following important concepts: metabolic rate, external versus internal sources of energy, and nutrients versus calories.

Feel Cold? Check Your Metabolic Rate

Most subjects on fairly severely calorie-restricted diets find that they are constantly cold even when dressed warmly. Humans are warm-blooded animals, which means they must keep their metabolic rate (the amount of energy the body uses in a given period) high enough to stay warm and keep the body's biochemical reactions humming along at the correct rate.

When your brain thinks you're starving, one of its first responses is to lower your metabolic rate in order to reduce your caloric requirements. The idea is that if you use less energy, you'll need fewer calories, which is a good thing if food is scarce. But having a low metabolic rate also makes you feel cold.

Notice that I said when your brain *thinks* you're starving. We'll find out that sometimes your brain thinks you're starving when you're not!

Food versus Stored Fat: External versus Internal Sources of Energy

The food you eat is your external source of energy. Your stored fat is your internal source of energy. Your brain can tell your body when to use this internal source, or—by making you feel hungry—when you need to use an external source (meaning eat more). Sometimes, however, even though your built-in pantry—that is, your belly—contains ample energy, your body is unable to access that energy, and therefore your brain senses a lack of nutrition and makes you feel hungry. So you eat more food rather than rely on your fat stores—not what you want to do if losing weight is your goal.

A Calorie Is a Calorie, Right? Nutrients versus Calories

If you compare the number of calories in the Keys and Hanssen diets, you'll see that they're similar: 1,570 and 1,850. However, if you compare the nutrients in the two diets, you'll notice a huge difference in the ratio of fats to carbohydrates. As you can see in the table that follows, the Hanssen diet contains about four times as much fat and eight times as many fat calories per carbohydrate calorie as the Keys diet (2.4 versus 0.3).

Name of Diet	Fat Calories	Carbohydrate Calories	Approximate Ratio of Fats to Carbohydrates	Hungry?
Keys Low-Fat Diet	17.2% (270 calories)	57.3% (900 calories)	0.3:1 (0.3 calories of fat for each calorie of carbohydrate)	Yes
Hanssen Higher-Fat Diet	60% (1,100 calories	25% (470 calories)	2.4:1 (2.4 calories of fat for each calorie of carbohydrate)	No

Table 3.2

The subjects on the Ancel Keys diet were hungry all the time, while those on the Per Hanssen diet were not. What about the cruise ship diet and the starvation diet? You would think that eating many more calories than your body requires would suppress appetite, while eating no calories would make you hungry. So why does the opposite happen? Let's compare the ratios of fats to carbohydrates and see what they suggest.

Name of Diet	Fat Calories	Carbohydrate Calories	Approximate Ratio of Fats to Carbohydrates	Hungry?
Cruise Ship	30% (1,350 calories)	50% (2,250 calories)	0.6:1 (0.6 calories of fat for each calorie of carbohydrate)	Yes
Starvation (calories burned are from internal sources)	70% (from internal stores)	20% (from internal stores)	3.5:1 (3.5 calories of fat for each calorie of carbohydrate)	No

Table 3.3

On the cruise ship diet, appetite increases in spite of eating excessive numbers of calories. However, during a brief period of total starvation, appetite decreases. This doesn't seem to make sense from the perspective of caloric intake. Just the opposite would be expected, namely, the people eating nothing should be hungrier than those aboard the cruise liner, who shouldn't be hungry at all.

However, could the nutrient content of the diet suggest an explanation? Hanssen's diet contained a high fat-to-carbohydrate ratio (2.4:1) that resembles the much higher starvation ratio of 3.5:1. Both of these seemed to be associated with less hunger. The cruise ship and Keys diets had low ratios (0.6:1 and 0.3:1, respectively), and the subjects on them were hungrier. This observation suggests that the *type* of calories you eat as well as the total number of calories consumed might make a difference in how your body responds to them, and this must be taken into consideration. A diet with a higher (and healthier) fat intake and a greater fat-to-carb ratio appears to be much more effective at producing satiety. Since you eat more when you are hungry, it seems as if the type of food that is consumed—in addition to its calorie content—makes a large difference in what you weigh.

Making Sense of the Diet Paradoxes

In this chapter I've described five diets—two low-calorie diets that produced opposite results, a starvation diet that suppressed appetite, a gluttonous diet that increased appetite, and a typical American diet. Let's see how what we've learned about insulin and its effect on fat cells explains these almost counterintuitive results.

The Keys Experiment

In the Keys experiment, healthy subjects were forced to eat a diet that was low in calories and low in fat. They lost weight but were cold and hungry all the time. The type of carbohydrates they ate kept their insulin levels high (making their fat cells sticky in the process). Because of that their fat stores were inaccessible. This, plus the fact that they were eating only about half the calories they usually did, made them feel ravenously hungry. Eating less food slowed their metabolism and made them feel cold. Ironically, obese people (whose "pantry" is even bigger) who follow similar diets also get hungry. Because their fat cells are sticky, they can't tap into the large amount of stored fat they carry around.

The Hanssen Experiment

The Hanssen subjects ate about the same number of calories as the Keys subjects, but they didn't feel hungry. Why? Because they were eating food with a higher fat-to-carb ratio that didn't substantially raise their insulin levels. As a result, their fat cells were able to release stored energy that prevented them from getting hungry and allowed them to lose weight in the process.

Total Starvation

When subjects eat no food at all, insulin levels plummet. Their fat cells become "un-sticky" and are able to release stored fat, thus providing all of the calories the brain and body need. So, in spite of eating no calories, no hunger develops.

Cruise Ship Eating

How can cruise ship guests eat so much and still be hungry all the time? The food they eat generates extremely high and persistently elevated insulin levels that keep their fat cells sticky. Consequently, a couple of hours after eating they feel hungry, eat again, and repeat this process over and over. So, in spite of eating many thousands of calories each day, they actually are hungrier than if they hadn't eaten anything at all.

The Typical American Diet

The typical American diet, which is filled with starchy vegetables like french fries, processed foods, snacks, and sugar-laden drinks, keeps insulin levels and hunger levels high much as the Keys diet did. You can see the result wherever you go in the United States—a shocking number of obese adults and children.

You now have the tools to think like a scientist. It's clear that not only *calories* count, but *what you eat* matters as well. In the next chapter we will meet John and Jane, who will help us understand how these concepts apply in "real-life" situations and why it's possible to eat like a bird and still gain weight.

4

CONTROLLING YOUR APPETITE BY FEEDING YOUR BRAIN

You might be wondering what the connection is between feeding your brain and controlling your appetite. Well, whether you are daydreaming about a certain food, feeling hungry, or just plain wanting to nosh, these are all brain states. There is an intimate connection among the brain, food, and the way we think about food. After all, from the brain's perspective, the body—including its ability to ambulate—is just a sophisticated conveyance designed to deliver food to the brain. Its appetite centers are merely the mechanism for making its feelings about food known.

You have probably noticed when you are hungry that it is not uncommon to have difficulty concentrating. When neurons in the appetite centers sense a lack of nutrients, they send out a hunger signal. Under similar conditions, neurons in other regions of the brain react as well. However, since they mediate different functions, such as focus and concentration, when they lack nutrients, symptoms like brain fog or mental fatigue appear. Nevertheless, in both circumstances the cause is identical: the brain has not been fed properly.

What Happens When You Eat?

Your body depends on two basic fuels for energy: carbohydrates (foods that are broken down into glucose) and fat. Depending upon what you have eaten and when, the fuel mixture your body burns at any point in time consists of a combination of both glucose and fat. However, the amount each contributes varies dramatically throughout the day. Right after a meal, glucose is the primary fuel. In between meals or while you are fasting—such as at night when you are asleep—the fuel mix contains a much higher fat content.

Also, when one fuel contributes more to the mixture being burned, the other plays a lesser role. So they both go through reciprocal peaks and valleys during a twenty-four-hour cycle. It sounds complicated, but the basics are pretty easy to understand.

As I mentioned in chapter 2, after a meal your blood glucose (blood "sugar") level rises and nourishes your body and brain. The presence of glucose in the blood also causes the insulin level to increase. Insulin controls blood sugar by transporting it out of the blood and into the cells of the body where it is burned up. This is why glucose is the primary source of energy when the insulin level rises after you eat.

At the same time, when insulin levels rise, fat gets sent into fat cells for storage—to be released after the carbohydrates that have just been eaten are used up. Thus, the rise and fall of insulin causes the fuel mixture to fluctuate between sugar and fat. In a sense, then, insulin functions as a nutrient-partitioning agent; you can think of it as a police officer who directs traffic one way or another. High insulin (which occurs after a meal) triggers fat storage and sugar burning. In between meals, when insulin is low, fat is released for use as a fuel source. If everything is in sync, these nutrients move back and forth providing the energy we need exactly when it is required. It's just that at certain times energy is generated from sugar while at other times energy is generated from fat.

Although every meal we consume has a different fat and carbohydrate composition, a similar overall response occurs each time we eat. Glucose is burned first while insulin is storing the fat that will be made available for use after the glucose is gone. It is the waxing and waning of the hormone insulin that coordinates this delicate process.

What should happen once the glucose and fat from the prior meal have been completely burned is that you start feeling hungry again. However, things don't always work as they are supposed to. To see what I mean, let's look at what happens to two people, John and Jane, after breakfast and how making the wrong food choices can produce disastrous results.

An Ideal Scenario: John's Morning

John starts to eat breakfast at 8:00. From shortly after 8:00 until about 9:30, his blood sugar level rises. This (appropriately) causes his insulin level to rise, which starts sugar burning while sending fat to be stored in his fat cells. By about 10:30, he has used up the initial rush of food energy from breakfast, his insulin level has decreased, and his fat cells release their stored energy for use as fuel for another couple of hours. Around noon, after both the initial food energy and the stored fat that was released are gone, he starts to feel hungry again.

Look at the following graph of the changes that occurred in John's body after breakfast. In figure 4.1 you will see two curves: one that depicts his glucose level (solid black), and one that charts his insulin level (dashed). During the interval depicted by the letter "A," he is in a fat-burning mode that started while he was sleeping the prior evening, a time when his insulin level was low. As his glucose and insulin levels begin to go up after breakfast (see the letter "B"), he starts burning

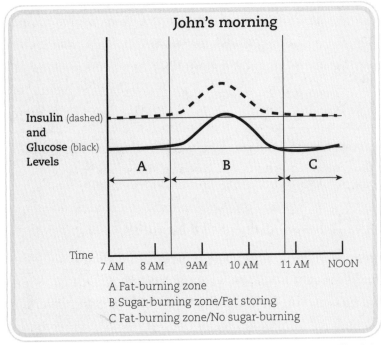

Fig. 4.1

glucose and simultaneously enters the fat-storing zone. This happens because his increasing insulin level activates the fat-storing switches on his fat cells.

At about 10:30, shown by the letter "C," John's glucose and insulin levels have fallen. This allows his fat cells to start releasing fat to burn for energy. The fat becomes the fuel source that carries him to lunchtime, when he becomes hungry again.

That's the ideal situation. However, as we saw in chapter 3, apparently not all calories are treated equally. To see what I mean, let's look at Jane's morning.

A Not-so-Ideal Scenario: Jane's Morning

Jane also began eating breakfast at 8:00. She and John are about the same size and eat the same number of calories. From 8:00 to 10:30, she uses some of the energy from the food she ate while an increasing insulin level directs her body to store the rest of it in her fat cells. So far it sounds just like John's morning. But at about 10:30, Jane starts feeling hungry again. Let's examine the graph (figure 4.2) and see what happened to her after breakfast. As shown by the letter "D," she began the day in a fat-burning mode that started the previous evening. After breakfast, because of the rise in insulin, she entered the sugar-burning and fat-storing mode (as John did), depicted by the letter "E." This continued until about 10:30 when, like John (see "F"), her blood sugar level had fallen back to normal and she left the sugar-burning zone. However, because of her persistently elevated insulin level (see the dashed insulin curve that is still elevated at 10:30), Jane was still in the fat-storing mode (see the shaded area under the insulin curve from 10:30 to noon). This is when she began to feel hungry. What made her appetite suddenly increase at 10:30 even though she ate the same number of calories as John? We'll explore that in detail in the next section.

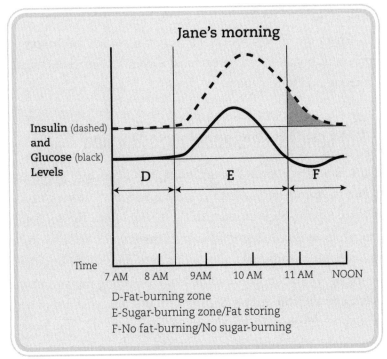

Fig. 4.2

Brain-Belly Basics

When insulin is high, fat gets sent into fat cells for storage.

What's the Difference Between These Two Scenarios?

Comparing figures 4.1 and 4.2 you can see that by about 10:30 the glucose level for both John and Jane has fallen back to its baseline value. The noticeable difference in the figures is that Jane's glucose curve peaked at a higher level than did John's, and she required more insulin (as shown by the higher insulin curve) to bring her glucose back down.

In addition, because of her higher glucose peak, Jane had an elevated insulin level that didn't return to normal until almost noon. (Compare her insulin level to John's.) It remained high *even after her blood sugar level returned to normal.* This persistently elevated insulin level kept her in a fat-storing mode for an extra ninety minutes (depicted by the shaded area under her insulin curve from 10:30 to 12:00). In contrast, John was back in a fat-burning mode again by 10:30 (when his insulin level had come back down to normal).

Jane, however, was prevented from tapping into her fat stores when she needed them at 10:30. Since she had essentially no access to fat or glucose from 10:30 on, she got hungry before John did. But the important question is: why did this happen?

It's time we examined what each of them ate for breakfast. (See tables 4.1 and 4.2.) As you can see, the number of calories was identical: 413. However, John's ratio of fat to carbohydrate calories was 1.9:1, while Jane's was much lower at 0.23:1. This means that he ate more fat and less carbohydrate than she did.

Since fat calories impact glucose and insulin levels minimally, it is no surprise that John's glucose and insulin levels were much lower than Jane's.

John's Breakfast Description (eaten as a mixture)	Calories	Carb Calories	Fat Calories	Protein Calories	Fat:Carb Ratio Calories
½ cup strawberries	25	21	0	4	
½ cup blueberries	42	38	1	3	
¾ cup cottage cheese	180	28	70	82	
¼ cup regular plain yogurt	38	12	18	8	
⅛ cup sliced almonds	68	4	51	13	
½ Tbsp. flax seed oil	60	0	60	0	
¼ tsp. ground cinnamon	0	0	0	0	
Total	413	103 (25%)	200 (48%)	110 (27%)	1.9:1

Table 4.1

In addition, the type of carbohydrates Jane chose to eat contained less fiber. By slowing down absorption, fiber blunts the rate at which glucose levels rise and subsequently prevents high insulin levels from developing. The presence of fiber in food is what makes it a slow release form of carbohydrate. Hence, the low fiber carbs she ate for breakfast were more rapidly absorbed and produced higher glucose and insulin levels.

Jane's Breakfast Description	Calories	Carb Calories	Fat Calories	Protein Calories	Fat:Carb Ratio Calories
1 cup corn flakes	100	91	0	9	
½ cup 2% fat milk	62	16	22	24	
1 cup orange juice	110	103	0	7	
1 slice whole wheat toast	65	40	9	16	
1 pat butter	36	0	36	0	
½ ounce grape jelly	40	40	0	0	
Total	413	290 (70%)	67(16%)	56 (14%)	0.23:1

Table 4.2

As depicted in Jane's graph, foods that stimulate a rapid and sustained rise in insulin eventually trick the body into thinking it is starving because the rise in insulin makes all the energy stores essentially invisible; hence, there is no fat or sugar burning (see figure 4.2, letter "F").

Most of us have plenty of stored fat—sometimes enough to last for several months. The problem is that it can't be released because the fat storage switch can't be turned off. This is precisely what happened to Jane and why she got hungry prematurely and had to eat again at 10:30.

I have chosen a man and a woman (John and Jane) to illustrate how what we eat is as important as how many calories we consume. The outcome would have been the same if two men or two women had been used in this example.

Foods That Fool Your Body

Jane got hungry as a result of prolonged, excessive, and unwanted fat storage. This happened because of the food choices she made during breakfast. As you can see in figure 4.2, when she needed to switch from using sugar to fat, her high insulin level prevented her from doing so.

She became hungry *even before her body had used up what she had just eaten*! So, by making the wrong food choices, she was "tricked" into eating again when she shouldn't have been hungry at all. And it had nothing to do with the number of calories she ate. The foods she chose for breakfast produced signals that were interpreted by her brain as hunger because of how the food was handled internally—that is, it was cleared from the circulation and placed in storage rather than remaining in the bloodstream for use by cells throughout the body.

Brain-Belly Basics

She became hungry even before her body had used up what she had just eaten!

It is no surprise that we can't survive without food. But because we have the ability to store food for use between meals, we don't have to eat continuously. Hormones are the chemical conductors that orchestrate the delicate process that determines how the energy from food is used. When they are in proper balance, the ebb and flow of nutrients are carefully regulated to provide a continual supply of energy that exactly matches our metabolic requirements. We are not prevented from running or being active simply because we haven't eaten and, likewise, we won't get hungry between meals.

> ## Brain-Belly Basics
>
> Hormones are the chemical conductors that orchestrate the delicate process that determines how the energy from food is used.

When hormones are doing their job properly, all is well. But how they work depends on the types of food choices we make. The interaction between food and hormones is an ancient one dating back millions of years. It evolved based on the body's responses to foods that were present during that era.

However, in recent times, eating habits have changed dramatically. About 80 percent of the food on the shelves of supermarkets today didn't exist a hundred years ago. Much of it is "manufactured" food that has been produced in factories rather than having been derived more directly from plants or animals.

To understand how this difference affects the body, let's look once more at what Jane ate for breakfast. Several foods—especially the corn flakes, OJ, and toast and jelly—triggered a large, prolonged surge of insulin because of the rapidly released carbohydrates they contain. This hormonal response was necessary to properly regulate Jane's blood glucose level. However, it takes the body a long time to bring such a high insulin level back down to normal. This excessive insulin surge keeps fat sequestered in fat cells at a time when the calories contained within them are needed to fuel the body. The result is a nutrient shortfall that is interpreted by the brain as impending starvation. This example illustrates how poor food choices can trick us into eating when our built-in pantries may be bursting with stored calories.

The take-home message is that Jane overate because she stored too much fat. She didn't gain weight because she ate too much (she ate the same number of calories as John, remember). This is an important distinction, because if she gained weight as the result of overeating, then the correct solution would be to eat less. However, she ate too much because she developed sticky fat cells. In this instance, *the appropriate response is to make proper food choices that prevent sticky fat cells from developing—not to eat less*. Non-sticky fat cells will then, in turn, prevent you from overeating.

> ## Brain-Belly Basics
> The appropriate response is to make proper food choices that prevent sticky fat cells from developing— not to eat less.

She Eats Like a Bird and Still Gains Weight!

Can this really happen? And if so, how can it possibly be explained? Let's see if we can make sense of this scenario using some of the principles discussed earlier.

If we haven't eaten in a while, hunger intensifies because the brain senses an impending food shortage. When insulin levels remain high, preventing us from accessing the fat stored in our bellies, this can also increase appetite. One occurs because of a shortage of "external" calories (food) and the other from a shortage of "internal" calories (stored fat).

If such conditions persist, the brain reacts by slowing down the rate at which calories are burned. This is what happens when people describe having a slow metabolism. It is how the body goes into "starvation mode," which allows it to survive longer using its fat stores. It was this process that allowed Helen Klaben and Ralph Flores to successfully endure their harrowing plane crash discussed in chapter 1. However, while a slower metabolism allows us to survive for a longer time when we are starving, it also means that it takes longer to burn fat and lose weight while dieting.

We are all familiar with people who ostensibly eat very few calories, are hungry all the time, and, in spite of this, gain weight. Whenever I was confronted with this scenario in the past, I found it difficult to believe. As a matter of fact, my initial reaction was that they were eating much more than they thought and that was the logical explanation for their weight gain.

We now have the tools to postulate another mechanism to explain how it might happen. Imagine someone eating a reduced calorie diet to lose weight. At first the pounds come off. Then a weight-loss plateau frequently occurs. One explanation for this is that the metabolic rate has slowed down and the number of calories being consumed just matches the number being burned—now a smaller number per day because of the slower metabolism.

To start the weight-loss process again, even fewer calories

must be consumed. After a while metabolism slows further and weight loss again sputters. The cycle must be repeated with even fewer calories. This is frequently how birdlike diets are initiated.

Now consider being on this type of diet and, in addition, mostly consuming foods that repeatedly spike insulin levels. These are bread, cookies, soda pop, and other comfort-type foods that will cause the calories being consumed to go directly to fat cells where they are stored rather than burned (because of the insulin spikes). In this example, if the number of calories being consumed is about 1,600 and 200 of them end up being

(For this exercise, assume that when you start out your body needs to burn 2,000 calories a day.)

Eating Like a Bird and Gaining Weight Diet	Feed Your Brain Lose Your Belly Diet
Cut calories to 1,800 per day and lose a bit of weight until a weight-loss plateau develops. Then cut calories to 1,600 per day to restart weight loss. If poor food choices are made (that generate high insulin levels), 200 of these calories are stored in fat, making only 1,400 calories available to burn. Now, the body goes into "starvation mode" and burns only 1,400 calories. This means 200 calories are stored as fat each day while eating like a bird.	Start eating 2,000 calories on the Feed Your Brain Lose Your Belly Diet. The low insulin level allows 300 calories of fat to be released from fat stores making 2,300 calories available to the body. This is more than it requires. Appetite eventually decreases, so soon you'll only need to consume 1,700 calories a day. Three hundred come from the released fat (to provide the 2,000 the body requires). Hence, 300 fat calories are lost each day and you don't get hungry.

locked in fat cells, it is really equivalent to eating only 1,400 calories since that is what the body has available to use. That is truly eating like a bird—a starving bird. Under these circumstances, metabolism slows drastically, possibly to the point where the body is burning only 1,400 calories in a twenty-four-hour period. This would mean that 200 calories are being stored each day, a situation in which weight is being gained while eating like a bird!

Hence, by restricting calories *and* making the wrong food choices, two things happen: metabolism slows, and we starve internally (meaning we store calories in fat cells where they are locked up and become inaccessible). Together, these conspire to enable us to store fat, gain weight, feel constantly hungry, and do so while on a starvation diet!

How is this situation to be avoided? First, don't start out by cutting calories. This merely serves as a signal for your metabolism to slow. Second, prevent the body from sending what you eat to fat cells for storage. The way to achieve this is by choosing foods that keep insulin levels low—slow-release carbohydrates, protein, and healthy fats. When you do this, your body makes the transition from burning external calories to burning internal calories—your fat stores. The result is that metabolism doesn't slow down, hunger doesn't develop, and fat cells shrink. This is what must be accomplished if weight loss is to be achieved.

If you know someone in this situation, do them a favor and tell them what to do about it!

Now it should be apparent that you don't get fat because you eat too many calories. You get fat because you've stored—and continue to store—too many calories as fat and can't access that fat when you need to. You're providing your brain and body with enough energy, but you're storing an excess amount of fat while doing so. For this reason, I call gaining weight a fat-storage problem. To see what I mean, look at the banking analogy that follows.

Banking Analogy

Suppose you have a job that pays you $1,000 every Friday. And every Friday you deposit $300 in a savings account while keeping $700 to spend for rent, food, gas, and so forth. Over the weekend, the bank is closed, and you can't withdraw money from your savings account. In effect, that $300 doesn't exist—it's as if you had been paid only $700.

The $300 in your savings account is like the calories you store in your fat cells, which are also unavailable for you to use. The difference is that on Monday you'll be able to withdraw your $300, whereas unless you start eating differently, the calories in your fat cells are permanently locked up!

What About Adult-Onset (Type 2) Diabetes?

It is important to understand the fundamental distinction between what happens in juvenile diabetes when sugar levels are high because no insulin can be produced and what typically occurs in Type 2 diabetes (usually seen in overweight people). In adults who are on the road to developing Type 2 diabetes, insulin levels are frequently quite high—much higher than normal—because of poor dietary choices. They stay elevated until the pancreas becomes unable to secrete the tremendous amounts of insulin that are required to control blood sugar levels. When this happens, adult-onset diabetes develops. Type 2 diabetics are usually overweight or obese and have elevated insulin levels. However, even though their insulin levels are quite high, they aren't able to produce enough insulin to regulate their blood sugar, so they need even more. This is why Type 2 diabetics often require insulin injections—to augment what their body is producing. However, when adult diabetics are put on insulin therapy, they usually gain weight, just as Jay Cutler did after he started insulin injections (see chapter 2).

Persons with Type 2 diabetes can decrease the amount of insulin they require by following the principles of the Feed Your Brain Lose Your Belly diet, but they should only consider cutting back on their insulin *under the close supervision of a physician*. Never do this on your own!

It All Adds Up!

By doing a little math, let's see how avoiding sticky fat cells can make a huge difference. For example, consider a typical healthy male who is 5'10" and weighs 150 pounds when he graduates from college at age twenty-two. Assume that he eats three meals and one snack a day. According to the U.S. Department of Agriculture (USDA) Economic Research Service (last updated 12/21/2004), the average American consumes 120 pounds of sugar/HFCS per year. That averages out to be about 150 grams (almost one-third of a pound!) per day, or a little less than 40 grams per meal for our "typical" subject.

This alone is sufficient to produce four fat-storing periods a day. If each contributes merely one gram of stored fat per meal, it adds up to four grams of fat storage per day. This is equivalent to thirty-six stored calories per day, or almost four pounds per year. What that means for this unlucky fellow is that by the time he reaches his thirty-second birthday, he will weigh an astounding 190 pounds! In just ten more years, he will weigh in at a portly 230 pounds as he hits middle age.

A quote attributed to Albert Einstein, the father of the modern theory of gravity, states, "The most powerful force in the universe is compound interest." Based on the above calculations I would suggest that the fat-storing power of insulin is a close second. The good news is that we can prevent our fat cells from becoming sticky by making the right food choices. How to make the proper food choices and what to eat will be discussed in detail in chapters 7 and 8.

FEED YOUR BRAIN . . . OR SUFFER THE CONSEQUENCES

Glucose is the primary fuel that sustains nerve cells. Since it can't store glucose, the brain is precariously dependent on a continuous supply in order to generate the energy it relies on to so deftly accomplish all the wonderful things it does for us. In addition, the brain is a real energy hog, burning fuel ten times faster than the rest of the body.

Insulin is the hormone whose job it is to keep blood sugar levels in the normal range. It performs this nifty task by transporting glucose from the blood into the muscles of the body. However, as insulin transports glucose into muscle cells, it *diverts it away from the brain.* This condition makes insulin's task somewhat tricky because it must keep the body happy without shortchanging the brain. As you have seen, insulin levels fluctuate during the course of a day. Hence, in the presence of too much insulin, the brain can suffer. Sophie's story illustrates in dramatic fashion how this tenuous balance can go awry.

Sophie's Story

The day started like any other Monday as Sophie woke up and eyed her alarm clock in the dim early morning light that filtered through her translucent drapes. She suddenly realized that she would be late for work yet again. While throwing on her clothes, hastily applying makeup, and grabbing her briefcase on the way out the door, her mind was on a meeting she would be leading at the end of the day. She slipped into the old Toyota 4Runner that had been a gift from her dad when she graduated from college and deftly guided it toward the on-ramp to I-70. The sun was low in the sky, and she was heading directly into it.

At about that time she began feeling somewhat lightheaded and woozy. Was this where she needed to turn? What a question for someone who had traveled the same route five days a week for the past twenty-two months. Oncoming cars appeared to be moving faster than she was used to. A vague, unsettling feeling was developing in the pit of her stomach, and it began to feel as if she were having an out-of-body experience. When a trickle of moisture appeared beneath her right armpit she realized that she was sweating, something she had never noticed before in the middle of winter.

In addition to that, a somewhat intangible nervousness had set in. This was a common occurrence when she had drunk too much coffee, but she didn't recall having had any this morning. The road appeared to be narrowing, and navigating between the closely spaced cars was becoming a chore. A simple trip to the office was beginning to feel like the Twilight Zone. Sophie's eyes were having trouble focusing, and her angst about being tardy for work started to feel unreal. Queasiness developed as the warmth of the heated car seat engulfed her.

The next thing Sophie knew, she was staring up into the eyes of a physician in the emergency room of the county hospital. It wasn't clear whether she was awake or if the whole thing was a dream. She was being asked to count backwards from ten, to squeeze the doctor's fingers, and to follow a flashlight with her eyes. "Are you taking any medications? Do you have any allergies? What is your health like?" are the questions she heard.

Not being fully coherent, she wasn't sure if she needed to respond or if the questions were directed at another person nearby. As her double vision cleared, it became apparent an IV tube was in her arm, and her vital signs were being monitored with electrical leads. A nurse came to her bedside and poked her finger with a needle to recheck her blood glucose level. As Sophie was dozing back to sleep, she was startled to hear, "Fifty-four. You're headed in the right direction!"

Now feeling more alert, Sophie asked what had happened to her. "You have diabetes, don't you?" the nurse asked.

"Well, yes," Sophie stammered.

"It seems like you overdid it with your medicine today. When you arrived, your blood sugar was about thirty, and you weren't making much sense. Luckily we identified that and started an IV to give you some sugar water. It did the trick; you look much better now. By the way, the paramedics said that when they arrived at the scene of the accident it looked like you had hit several cars and had come to rest in a large hedge. It was fortunate that nobody was injured."

Startled, Sophie responded: "Nothing like this has ever

happened to me before. The funny part is that I don't remember a thing! I know I was in a hurry as I left for work, and I must have taken too much insulin."

"You're going to be fine. But we'll have to watch you for a while to make sure your blood tests stabilize. However, we'll need to have a family member drive you home later in the day," said the nurse.

Too Much of a Good Thing

This scenario is played out with some regularity in many ERs throughout the country. What happened to Sophie is a typical result that illustrates an important lesson. *Too much insulin is bad for the brain.*

> ### Brain-Belly Basics
> Too much insulin is bad for the brain.

In people who don't have diabetes, blood glucose levels fluctuate throughout the day in relation to the types and amounts of food that are consumed. Diets that contain more sugar and foods that are rapidly broken down into glucose cause blood glucose levels to rise. When this happens, the body's response is to release more insulin. The greater the rise in blood glucose, the higher the insulin goes.

Problems arise when "spikes," or dramatic rises, in the level of insulin occur. They can produce subsequent periods of hypoglycemia (low blood sugar) because the insulin stays in the bloodstream longer than glucose, and it subsequently tends to drive glucose levels below normal. (Look back at figure 4.2 and see that Jane's glucose level went below normal at about 10:30.) If these swings are mild, you might only feel hungry. When they are more severe, it is not uncommon to feel shaky or jittery or to develop brain fog and not think clearly. When insulin levels are persistently elevated, or in people with blood sugar regulating problems, brain problems can be even more severe.

As you can see, what we eat determines how much insulin is released. In diabetics like Sophie, who can't make any insulin because she developed juvenile diabetes, several daily insulin injections are required. They need to guess how much glucose-rich (meaning carbohydrate-containing) food will be consumed at a given meal and then calculate how much insulin to inject to "cover" the expected rise in blood sugar the meal will produce. If insufficient insulin is administered, blood glucose levels remain elevated. If too much is given, glucose levels fall, sometimes so low that they cause the type of symptoms Sophie experienced.

Less dramatic swings in blood sugar can occur in people who don't have diabetes. They are usually caused by sugar binges followed shortly thereafter by a large insulin spike. However, as is evident, too much insulin—whether injected or in conjunction with poor dietary choices—can contribute to brain starvation.

Effect of Elevated Insulin on the Brain

As Sophie learned, when insulin levels are high, glucose (the brain's main fuel) is directed away from the brain and into other tissues, such as muscle. As was discussed previously, persistently elevated insulin also keeps fat locked in fat cells.

This combination makes us fat and starves our brains by diverting nutrients away from neurons and into other cells for storage. While swings in insulin might not be as dramatic in non-diabetic individuals, they occur nonetheless, and can make us hungry and contribute to brain aging and even more ominous problems.

Brain-Belly Basics

Too much insulin can contribute to brain starvation.

This is easily demonstrated by looking at statistics relating disorders of glucose and insulin metabolism to the incidence of the major neurodegenerative disorder being seen throughout the world—Alzheimer's disease. Diabetics have four times the risk for developing Alzheimer's; those with prediabetes have triple the risk, and persons with pre-prediabetes (meaning that their blood sugar is normal all the time, but they have to work harder to control it by releasing more insulin throughout the day) have double the risk. These are a few of the reasons why many brain scientists around the world are beginning to refer to Alzheimer's disease as Type 3 diabetes. In Type 1 and Type 2 diabetes, there is an inability to efficiently use glucose throughout the body. Type 3 diabetes refers to the same problem in the brain—with the ominous consequences just discussed.

How to Prevent Alzheimer's Disease

Over the past ten years, neuroscientists have identified an inability of the brain in Alzheimer's patients to properly use glucose. This has been documented by sensitive brain scans called positron emission tomography, or PET, scans. In certain instances, these changes can be seen decades before a diagnosis of Alzheimer's disease is made, which suggests to experts in this field that the inability of the brain to properly use glucose might be a key factor in the development of the disease.

A recent paper published in the journal *Archives of Neurology* by Suzanne Craft and her associates has even identified these ominous PET scan findings in subjects with diabetes and prediabetes. This observation led the researchers to believe that these conditions were risk factors for the development of Alzheimer's disease.

To prevent diabetes of the brain and the body, it makes sense to select foods that feed the brain while maintaining stable blood sugar and insulin levels. In Part 2 of *Feed Your Brain, Lose Your Belly* you'll learn exactly how to accomplish this.

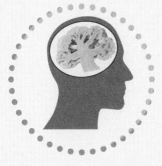

PART 2

The Feed Your Brain Lose Your
Belly Diet and Activity Program

DEMONIZED FAT: ESSENTIAL FOR BRAIN AND BODY WELLNESS

On Friday, January 14, 1977, Senator George McGovern announced the publication of the first *Dietary Goals for the United States*. He called them "the first comprehensive statement by any branch of the federal government on risk factors in the American diet." It was also the first time the government had sent a message to all Americans that they could better their health by eating less fat. Their intention was to diminish the fat content of the diet from approximately 40 percent, what it was at the time, to 30 percent. Although the *Dietary Goals* admitted the existence of a scientific dietary controversy regarding their sweeping recommendations, it was insisted that Americans had nothing to lose by following them.

The government was strikingly successful in achieving its objective. Current fat intake is about 30 percent of calories consumed. However, if one examines obesity statistics compiled by the Centers for Disease Control over the ensuing years, there has been a progressive rise in the number of obese children and adults. Adult and childhood obesity have more than doubled since the *Dietary Goals* were announced. This bears repeating: a 100 percent increase in obesity that correlated with a 10 percent decrease in fat content in the diet. Although calorie consumption has increased a bit, it alone cannot account for the obesity epidemic we are experiencing today.

Included in the most recent (2010) dietary recommendations from the United States Department of Agriculture (USDA) are additional impassioned pleas to purge still more fat from our plates—recommendations inextricably linked with a reciprocal increase in carbohydrate calories in the diet. Given the soaring obesity rates, the committee that approves the recommendations must be thinking they haven't restricted fat enough to make us all thin.

To further muddy the waters, the USDA is charged with both supporting farmers and advising Americans about what to eat. The same USDA that pays farmers billions of dollars in farm subsidies to grow corn, wheat, and rice—and thereby produce the ocean of high-fructose corn syrup we are drowning in—"recommends" all of these same foods in *My Food Pyramid*, apparently still believing Americans have nothing left to lose by consuming them. Corn is even doubly recommended, listed as it is in two food groups—grains and vegetables. Some would consider this a conflict of interest, encouraging Americans to eat just what the farmers are being paid to grow.

The *Dietary Goals* justified its recommendations, in part based on the assumption that the lower percentage of fat calories in the diet would make weight gain less likely—allegedly due to the higher caloric density of fat. What have not been adequately considered in this proposal are the adverse hormonal impacts of the coincident increase in carbohydrate consumption and the loss of the beneficial effects of fat in the diet. I have intensively discussed the carbohydrate-insulin link. Now I will take on the myth that has marginalized dietary fat consumption.

If it were true that eating too much is the only thing that makes you get fat, then consciously restricting food intake might make sense. But, as we've seen by investigating the food choices of John and Jane, the real problem is the development of sticky fat cells. High insulin levels are the driver behind the sticky fat cell problem, and the amount and type of carbohydrates in the diet determine how much insulin is produced. So, making food choices that avoid the production of sticky fat cells, rather than forcing ourselves to eat less, is the best way to stay thin and prevent calories from bypassing hungry brain cells. Including healthy fats in the diet also contributes to keeping fat cells from getting sticky.

Brain-Belly Basics

So, making food choices that avoid the production of sticky fat cells, rather than forcing ourselves to eat less, is the best way to stay thin and prevent calories from bypassing hungry brain cells.

Foods that elevate glucose and insulin levels are ranked by their propensity to do so in glycemic index tables. Fats are not included in these tabulations. Why? Because they don't raise glucose and insulin levels. Hence, *dietary fats don't contribute to the sticky fat cell problem*. In addition, as was seen in the Hanssen diet, fats profoundly decrease appetite. Anything that decreases appetite and avoids sticky fat cells should be included in the diet. Later in this chapter we will see why incorporating more healthy fats is also a brain-saver.

Brain-Belly Basics

Dietary fats don't contribute to the sticky fat cell problem.

Eat Fat to Lose Fat?

At this point you may be thinking: "It's all so confusing. If I want to get rid of fat, why is eating additional fat going to make me thinner? Won't I have to burn the fat that I eat plus what I'm already carrying around?"

The simple answer to that question is "yes." But to see why eating fat to lose fat makes sense, you must understand how fat is handled and how the hormonal changes that are induced actually produce weight loss. As was already discussed, fat in the diet doesn't increase the level of insulin floating around in the blood. So eating more fat (while consuming the same number of calories) simultaneously provides the body with a wonderful fuel source and avoids the sticky fat cell problem.

Why does this approach speed up weight loss? Because it allows us to rely more on calories stored in our fat cells and less on calories in the foods we eat. Basically, we start to burn internal (stored) rather than external (eaten) calories. As we make this transition (which must happen if weight is to be lost), we spontaneously eat less because a larger proportion of the calories being burned comes from our fat stores.

To put things another way, eating like this facilitates the metabolic transition that enables us to burn more stored fat by diminishing appetite (as demonstrated in the dietary analysis presented in chapter 4). As hunger decreases, the body naturally relies more on internal energy than on what we eat, which results in weight loss. When this happens without increasing appetite, diets are easy to stick to long-term.

> ## Brain-Belly Basics
>
> Eat more of the right fats and select foods that act as slow-release carb sources. This will dramatically curb your appetite.

Is There Such a Thing as Healthy Fat?

If we ate no fat in our diet, we would develop what is referred to as a dietary deficiency disease. For example, a diet that contains no thiamin (a B vitamin) leads to the development of a disorder called beriberi (vitamin B1 deficiency) since B vitamins are essential nutrients in our diet. Because our body can't make these essential nutrients, we must consume them each day or suffer the consequences.

There is an array of nutrients for which this is the case. They include vitamins (both fat and water soluble), certain amino acids (protein building blocks), minerals (such as calcium and magnesium), and certain other micronutrients, including manganese, iron, selenium, and chromium and many others. You might notice that there are no "essential" carbohydrates. Just as there are essential amino acids that our body can't make, there are also essential fats (called fatty acids) that fall into the same category. Hence, they must be included in the diet or a deficiency disease will develop. For this reason, they are referred to as essential fats, and they include two main categories: linoleic acid, an omega-6 type of fat, and α-linolenic acid, an omega-3 type of fat. Two related subcategories of these two essential fats—their long-chain cousins, if you will—are equally important: arachidonic acid, an omega-6 fat found in meat, and the omega-3 fat docosahexaenoic acid (DHA) found in coldwater fish. If these essential fats are not included in our diets, we will get sick.

As a matter of fact, the omega-3 fats are so important that many experts in the field of child development believe that omega-3 fatty acid deficiency is a contributor to the epidemic of ADD/ADHD we are currently experiencing. Fat is not only essential, it is vital for the proper functioning of our most important organs.

In addition to the essential fats, many other types of fats play indispensable roles throughout our bodies. These are called *functional fats* because of the important metabolic tasks they perform and *structural fats* due to the contribution they make to the composition of our cells and organelles (special compartments within cells).

Other types of fats are primarily stored in our fat cells as buffers against food shortages. There are even special types of fats that are preferentially burned rather than stored, thus keeping our energy levels up. You have probably not heard much about this last category of special fats, but you will shortly.

Why Limit Fat?

If fat is so important, why have we been told for years to limit the amount of fat we eat? Good question! One possible answer is that if we want to lose fat, then we should eat less of it. The problem with this approach is the adverse hormonal impact of doing so. In addition, we have all witnessed the disastrous impact of eating a low-fat diet on our waistlines and know we must move on.

Each day, fascinating nutritional information becomes available that enables us to make better decisions about what to eat. For example, many of the older guidelines didn't factor in the inflammatory responses generated by the foods that were being recommended at the time. We are now aware of the central role inflammation plays in heart disease, joint and bone degeneration, and brain disorders. Healthy fats and colorful fruits and vegetables decrease inflammation in the body and should be incorporated into any healthy diet.

Different Types of Fat

Just as carbohydrates are not all created equal, the same applies to fats. One type should be avoided at all costs. It is a category called *trans fats* and is listed collectively under the name *partially hydrogenated oils*. On food labels, they typically appear as partially hydrogenated corn oil, partially hydrogenated sunflower oil, or partially hydrogenated safflower oil. Food manufacturers use these man-made fats to extend the shelf life of packaged goods. The only problem is that they are unhealthy and can elevate LDL cholesterol (the "bad" cholesterol) and lower HDL cholesterol (the "good" cholesterol).

Not only are they bad for heart health, they are also bad for the brain because they counteract the beneficial actions of the healthy omega-3 fats. For these reasons, trans fats should be on your list of foods to avoid completely. However, you need to read labels carefully to see where they are lurking. They are in everything from french fries to cookies. Trans fats may even contribute to weight gain, based on findings in a six-year-long study in monkeys fed a diet containing them.

The other type of fat that should be minimized is animal fat that occurs in the form of the white, lard-like portion of roasts. It is basically a collection of (primarily) long-chain saturated fat molecules—a form of empty calories—that is similar to what we store in our pantries. It can easily be trimmed, although leaving a bit of it adds to the flavor of the meat when it is cooked.

While intrinsically not too bad, animal fat is a source of calories without much nutritional benefit, so why eat a lot of it in the first place? Having noted that, I'd like to mention a couple of its beneficial attributes, including the ability to elevate HDL cholesterol (the "good" cholesterol). It is also one of the few ways to lower lipoprotein(a), a potent risk factor for heart disease—something that no medications currently on the market can accomplish.

The Importance of "Balance"

The two types of essential fats—omega-6 and omega-3—are available in many foods. The problem is that they should be balanced in our diet, which means that they must be consumed in roughly equal amounts to keep their ratio close to 1:1. What has happened, largely due to the prevalence of vegetable oils on grocery store shelves, is that we eat far too much omega-6 fat and not enough omega-3. The impact of this dietary imbalance has produced omega-6/omega-3 ratios in the 20:1 range, which induces unhealthy inflammatory changes in our bodies

Omega-6 fat sources	
Safflower oil	
Sunflower oil	
Corn oil	
Soybean oil	
Nuts	
Seeds	
Omega-3 fat sources	
Salmon	Mackerel
Herring	Wild game such as venison
Sardines	and buffalo
Halibut	Flax seeds
Anchovies	Flax seed oil
Bluefish	Walnuts
Tuna	Leafy greens
	Hemp seed oil
	Purslane

Note: Soy and flax contain plant-based components that can affect hormonal signaling in the body. These pathways potentially involve estrogen, progesterone, and thyroid hormones. Please check with your health-care practitioner to see what is recommended for you.

Table 6.1

Content of Long-Chain Omega-3 Fat (grams) per 100-Gram Serving (about 3.5 ounces)

Atlantic Salmon (farmed)	1.8	Pollock	0.5
Anchovy (canned in oil)	1.7	Oyster	0.5
Sardine	1.4	Halibut	0.4
Herring (pickled)	1.2	Scallop	0.3
Mackerel	1.0	Shrimp	0.3
Trout (Rainbow, farmed)	1.0	Haddock	0.2
Swordfish	0.7	Clam	0.2
Tuna (white, canned in water)	0.7	Cod	0.1
Mussel (blue)	0.7		

Source: USDA Nutrient Database for Standard Reference

Table 6.2

Content of Shorter-Chain Omega-3 Fat (grams) per 1-Ounce Serving: Nuts and Seeds

Walnuts	2.6	Poppy seeds	0.1
Flax seeds	1.8	Pumpkin seeds (shelled)	0.1
Pecans (dry roasted)	0.3	Sesame seeds	0.1
Pistachios (roasted)	0.1	Almonds (dry roasted)	0.0

Source: Minnesota Nutrient Database 4.04 (last revised 3/02)

Table 6.3

Content of Shorter-Chain Omega-3 Fat (grams) per 1-Tablespoon Serving

Flax seed oil	6.9	Soybean oil (unhydrogenated)	0.9
Walnut oil	1.4		
Canola oil	1.3	Olive oil	0.1

Source: Minnesota Nutrient Database 4.04 (last revised 3/02)

Table 6.4

Content of Shorter-Chain Omega-3 Fat (grams) per 1-Cup Serving	
Spinach (fresh, cooked). . . 0.2	Collard greens (cooked). . . 0.2
Dandelion greens (cooked) 0.2	Green leaf lettuce . . . . . trace
Kale (cooked) 0.2	

Source: Minnesota Nutrient Database 4.04 (last revised 3/02)

Table 6.5

and may contribute to making us fatter. To normalize the ratio of essential fats we must markedly diminish omega-6 intake (see table 6.1) and enhance omega-3 consumption (see also tables 6.2, 6.3, 6.4, and 6.5).

MUFAs

Monounsaturated fat (see table 6.6) is a very healthy type of fat. It is a liquid at room temperature and becomes thicker or even semi-solid when refrigerated. Olive oil is a common example of oil that contains monounsaturated fatty acids (MUFAs). MUFAs help lower "bad" cholesterol without affecting levels of "good" cholesterol.

They can even speed up belly fat loss. In one study, dieters who consumed MUFAs lost 56 percent more central body fat than those on a low-fat diet. And this was accomplished without cutting calories or doing additional exercise! Findings in another study showed that a meal containing MUFAs enhanced fat-burning for the next five hours.

MUFAs also help normalize blood sugar levels—in a very unusual manner. When intake of MUFAs is increased, the body produces more of a hormone called adiponectin. Higher levels of it are beneficial because adiponectin improves glucose metabolism.

Good MUFA Sources		
Oils (1 Tbsp contains 120 calories)	**Nuts** (½ oz)	**Other**
Flax oil Olive oil Sesame oil Walnut oil	Almonds, 82 cal. Brazil nuts, 85 cal. Cashews (dry roasted), 82 cal. Hazelnuts, 79 cal. Macadamias (dry roasted), 101 cal. Pistachios (dry roasted), 80 cal. Walnuts, 92 cal.	¼ medium avocado, 70 cal. ½ oz dark chocolate, 75 cal. 1 olive, 10 cal.

Table 6.6

Coconut—The Miracle Oil!

The numerous benefits of coconut oil are finally being recognized. They include its unique ability to promote a healthy metabolism and provide almost immediate energy. In addition, it is the best cooking oil on the planet! Olive oil is good, but coconut oil is truly superb. Its delicate taste will enhance anything you are cooking, and it is not damaged by heat.

You might hear people say that coconut oil contains the most saturated fat of any edible oil. But not all saturated fats are created equal. They come in different lengths. Long-chain saturated fats are primarily stored in fat tissue throughout the body.

Most of the fats in coconut oil, however, are medium-chain lengths and are called medium-chain triglycerides (MCTs). When they are eaten, they go directly to the liver, where they are converted into a readily available energy source rather than being stored as fat. In fact, the MCTs in coconut oil can actually stimulate your metabolism, leading to weight loss!

This was discovered serendipitously back in the 1940s when farmers tried to use inexpensive coconut oil to fatten their livestock. To their surprise, the cattle became leaner, not fatter. Since then, numerous studies have shown that you lose weight when you replace long-chain fat (saturated or unsaturated) in your diet with the same amount of medium-chain fat.

The MCTs in coconut oil are metabolized into compounds called ketone bodies, also known as ketones. We will see how ketones are brain-savers and can be used easily by neurons to decrease appetite and sharpen focus, memory, and concentration.

The bottom line is to add coconut oil to your diet for all these reasons. It is available in most grocery stores, although many clerks may not know which aisle it is in. It is also available online.

Ketones and the Brain–Belly Connection

Usually only DHA is mentioned when one discusses omega-3 fatty acids and brain health. This is because it keeps the membranes of our nerve cells soft and flexible, traits that allow them to be exquisitely responsive to the trillions of signals they must process. Make no mistake: DHA is vital for a sharp mind. However, based on recent findings from Dr. Stephen Cunnane, a noted Canadian expert on diet and nutrition, other omega-3 fats are just as important. DHA's shorter relative—α-linolenic acid—another omega-3 fat, must now be visualized from an entirely new perspective. In addition to being a precursor for DHA (meaning it can be chemically transformed into DHA by the body), it is also able to be metabolized into ketones, as Dr. Cunnane's novel observations have demonstrated.

What are ketones, and why is this discovery noteworthy? Remember, the primary fuel for neurons is glucose. When not enough of it is available, the brain stops working. We saw this demonstrated tellingly when Sophie wound up in the ER from hypoglycemia caused by her insulin overdose. Fat, protein, and carbohydrate can be used as fuel for the body. However, of the three, only glucose (what carbohydrates are broken down into) can be used by the brain. The good news is that ketones provide an additional fuel source for nerve cells, which our brains are full of. The not-quite-good news is that ketones are not available in grocery stores—directly.

When fats are partially oxidized (science-speak for what happens when fats are burned in cells), ketones can be generated. This happens very easily to α-linolenic acid. Stated differently, α-linolenic acid is very ketogenic. That means it produces ketones in the body. So, foods that contain α-linolenic acid are the source of a powerful brain fuel, and an additional energy source—one that is even higher octane than glucose! Whenever glucose is in short supply, ketones can fill in. Sources of α-linolenic acid are listed in tables 6.1, 6.3, 6.4, and 6.5.

It might be helpful to provide an example of why having an optional energy source (ketones) in addition to glucose is important. Since the brain doesn't care where its energy comes from (glucose or ketones), when glucose is in short supply, ketones can easily fill in. It's like hybrid cars being able to use ethanol instead of gasoline. The use of glucose and ketones in the brain is an analogous situation. This beneficial action might have been helpful for Sophie when she was taken to the ER suffering from hypoglycemia. She lost consciousness because there was insufficient glucose to produce all the energy the brain required. If ketones had been present, they could have been a substitute fuel for the neurons. When this happens, there is no power shortage, and no symptoms of brain starvation develop.

Ketones can also be used by neurons under somewhat different circumstances to sharpen focus, memory, and concentration. To underscore how effective this approach is, let's consider the product Axona. Axona is considered to be a medical food. There are very few medical foods on the market. Products in this unique category require a prescription but are not drugs. They are consumable foods or beverages that are used for the treatment of diseases. The disease Axona treats is moderate and severe Alzheimer's disease. It can frequently be used with any of the other Alzheimer drugs on the market because it works in a different manner. It allows the brain cells to generate more energy and hence function better. It performs this miraculous feat by producing large amounts of brain-friendly ketones!

Because ketones can be used by any nerve cells, when they are taken up in the appetite centers of the brain, appetite decreases. This novel property is important because it is another reason why fats, especially those that generate ketones, play a central role in weight control.

Other Sources of Ketones

In addition to including coconut oil and the universe of omega-3 foods containing α-linolenic acid in your diet, there are other simple ways to increase the ability of your body to generate ketones internally. Not surprisingly, they are part of the Feed Your Brain Lose Your Belly diet. Because ketones are generated when fat is being burned in the liver, anything that facilitates fat burning will generate more ketones.

Ketones are naturally present in abundance during periods of starvation. This is a time when we rely almost exclusively on fat from our built-in pantries. During prolonged food shortages, insulin levels fall for this very reason. So, eating to minimize insulin production, in addition to all of its other health benefits, naturally stimulates ketone formation. This approach involves choosing the right carbohydrates—those that are slowly digested and produce minimal blood sugar fluctuations. These are usually the ones with higher fiber content. We will get into the nuts and bolts of which ones they are shortly.

MAKING THE BEST FOOD CHOICES

The Feed Your Brain Lose Your Belly diet doesn't require you to weigh, measure, or count what you eat. It relies on making food choices that prevent the development of sticky fat cells. This, in turn, has a potent appetite suppressant effect. You will *naturally* eat less because you are burning more stored calories.

Brain-Belly Basics

You will naturally eat less because you are burning more stored calories.

When you make the proper food choices, how much you eat takes care of itself. As you enjoy meals containing high-quality lean protein and healthy fats, along with nutrient- and fiber-rich foods, you'll have little desire to overeat. On this program, you'll get in touch with your body and be able to distinguish between *feeling hungry* and merely *wanting to eat*. Likewise, you'll recognize emotional eating, eating because you're depressed or bored, and eating just for the sake of eating. Once you become attuned to the sometimes subtle signals you will be receiving, you'll eat only what you need. However, it doesn't mean that calories don't count. For this reason, to provide guidance when you are first starting, I have made suggestions about portion sizes to be used for the more calorie-dense foods in the fats and oil categories. When you experience how effective even small amounts of fatty foods are at restraining appetite, you will no longer need to measure their serving sizes.

As a rough guide, I recommend that roughly 20 percent of daily calories come from protein and that about 15–25 percent come from carbohydrates. The remaining 55–65 percent of daily calorie content comes from fat. Remember that these are approximate guidelines, not rigid mandates. We're all different, and amounts and quantities can vary from day to day. The food choices you make are more important than the exact proportions.

To get started, I suggest that you include lean protein, slow-release carb choices, and herbs and spices with each meal. Try to incorporate five servings (⅔ cup) of veggies and two servings from the fruit (½ cup) category each day.

Eat good fats at each meal. Choose primarily from the monounsaturated fat group. Also try to include sources of coldwater fish containing long-chain omega-3 fat several times a week. Add flax seeds or flax oil every day. Get creative about the use of coconut oil.

For example, at breakfast add one or two tablespoons of coconut oil and a tablespoonful of flax seed oil to a bowl of cooked steel cut oats sprinkled with cinnamon and topped with strawberries. Add a delicious hard-boiled egg. For lunch, mix ½ tablespoon of flax seed oil with 1-½ tablespoons of olive oil and some balsamic vinegar, salt, pepper, and fennel and serve over a mixed green salad. Savor a small handful of nuts (fifteen), several small squares of cheese, and a few grapes for an afternoon snack. Combine three or four avocado slices with some rosemary chicken and asparagus with a drizzle of butter and fresh dill for dinner.

See table 7.1 for the good carbs to choose from and table 7.2 for the bad carbs to minimize. Be creative. Make selections you haven't tried before. Experiment with an array of colors, shapes, and sizes. Strive to make the food look as good as it tastes. Choose fruits and veggies from many cultures! Don't forget the herbs and spices, which are virtually calorie free and contain an almost endless supply of valuable phytonutrients such as antioxidants (free-radical fighters) and anti-inflammatories. Spend time learning how to combine them in unexpected ways. Doing so can dramatically alter the taste of a dish that has become boring. Mix spicy and sharp with sweet and mild. Use coconut oil for cooking, and add it to other dishes for its delicate flavor.

Table 7.3 includes a brief, practical listing of the generally available plant-based fat sources (with the inclusion of butter). Try to incorporate two or three servings from the nuts and seeds category each day. Olive oil is a good source of MUFAs. So is macadamia nut oil. It is just not as widely available. I use the polyunsaturated vegetable oils sparingly because of their

Good Carbs

Vegetables	Legumes	Fruit
(Good slow-release carbohydrates)	Black beans	(Note: fruit can be high in sugar content so I suggest 2 servings per day with sizes as shown below.)
Artichoke hearts	Black-eyed peas	Apple, 1
Arugula	Broad beans	Apricots, 4 fresh or 6 dried
Asparagus	Butter beans	Banana, ½
Bok choi	Chickpeas (garbanzos)	Blackberries, ½ cup
Broccoli	Edamame	Blueberries, ½ cup
Brussels sprouts	Italian beans	Cantaloupe, 1 small slice
Cabbage	Kidney beans	Cherries, 15
Cauliflower	Lentils	Clementine, 1
Celery	Lima beans	Cranberries, ½ cup
Chard	Navy beans	Grapefruit, ¼
Collard greens	Pinto beans	Grapes, 10
Cucumbers	Soybeans	Honeydew, 1 small slice
Eggplant		Kiwi, ½
Endive		Mango, ⅙
Green and yellow beans		Nectarine, ½
Hearts of palm		Orange, 1
Jicama		Peach, ½
Kale		Pear, ¼
Kohlrabi		Plum, 1
Leeks		Prune, 2
Lettuce		Raspberries, ½ cup
Mushrooms		Strawberries, ½ cup
Okra		Tangerine, 1
Onions		
Peppers		
Radishes		
Scallions		
Shallots		
Spinach		
Squash		
Tomatoes		
Turnip greens		
Watercress		

Table 7.1

Bad Carbs

(Limit or avoid entirely)	Artificial Sweeteners
Bread	(Use sparingly)
Cake	Acesulfame K
Candy	Aspartame (NutraSweet,
Cookies	Equal)
Corn	Saccharin
Dates	(Sweet'N Low)
Figs	Sucralose
High fructose corn syrup (HFCS)	(Splenda)
Honey	
Ice cream	
Jam and jelly	
Pasta (OK in small amounts, al dente is better)	
Rice	
Rolls	
Soda	
Sugar	
Watermelon	
White or red potatoes	

Table 7.2

high omega-6 content. They are not good cooking oils because of their polyunsaturated composition. Flax seed oil is not a good choice for cooking for the same reason. I prefer to cook with coconut oil, butter, and olive oil. Include two or three servings from the flax and coconut oil group each day. These tend to be foods that have been blacklisted because of their fat content. As you reintroduce them into your diet, I hope your palate enjoys them as much as mine does.

Some people enjoy meat more than others. I don't necessarily choose the leaner cuts. Some fat can make a steak taste more sumptuous. The game meats are usually quite lean and might require adding fat to any dishes containing them. Some

Nuts, Seeds, Oils, and Other Fats

Remember that these are calorie-dense foods. Numbers are suggested serving sizes. Two to three servings of nuts or seeds are recommended per day.

Nuts and Seeds	Oils	Other Fats
Almonds. 15	**MUFA-containing oils**	Avocado (¼ to ½ whole or 1 Tbsp oil)
Brazil nuts 4	• Canola	
Cashews. 15	• Olive	Butter (1 or 2 pats per day)
Filberts 20	**Products containing polyunsaturated oils**	
Flax seed . . 3 Tbsp	(Use sparingly)	Margarine (trans fat free, 1 or 2 pats per day)
Hazelnuts. 20	• Corn	
Macadamia nuts . 9	• Peanut	
Pecans. 12	• Safflower	Olives (5–10, or ½ Tbsp oil) (If in salad dressing, use 2 Tbsp)
Pine nuts . . . . .1 oz	• Sesame	
Pistachios 25	• Soybean	
Pumpkin seeds. . . . . . 3 Tbsp	• Sunflower	
Sesame seeds. . . . . . 3 Tbsp	**Specialty Oils** (Try to include 1 or 2 Tbsp per day of each)	
Sunflower seeds. . . . . . .3 Tbsp	• Coconut (an excellent cooking oil)	
Walnuts 15	• Flax seed	

Table 7.3

people find that chicken tends to be easier to digest. Soy-based products can be high in protein, and I have tasted some real soy delicacies in vegetarian restaurants. Although they are not listed in table 7.4, eggs are an excellent food and a great protein source.

A discussion of the glycemic index (GI) concept will help you make better carb choices. The GI is a number assigned to foods that contain carbohydrates—remember, they are the triggers that raise glucose and insulin levels. This number helps guide food choices by providing a relative rating scale that reflects the impact of each food on blood sugar. (Note that fat and protein don't impact blood sugar and are not on the GI list.)

The GI is determined by feeding humans who have fasted overnight a 50-gram portion of the desired food. Blood samples are then drawn every fifteen minutes for three hours. These values are plotted on a graph. The resultant curve reflects the impact of that food on subsequent blood sugar levels. It is then compared with the graph obtained after a 50-gram glucose meal, which is rated arbitrarily as being 100. Generally speaking, the lower the GI rating, the lower the impact of the food on blood glucose levels. Numbers over 70 are high, those under 55 are better, and those below 30 are very good.

The GI of each food that contains carbohydrates has been calculated. For example, glucose is rated at 100. Corn flakes are 98. A French baguette is 95. A baked potato is 93. Whole wheat bread is 77. A donut is 76. Popcorn is 72. Pizza is 60. Raisins are 56. Strawberries are 42. Lentils are 30. Cherries are 22. Broccoli is 10. Table 7.5 shows a more complete listing of the GI of a number of everyday foods.

Meat, Seafood, Cheese, and Dairy

Beef	Poultry	Cheese
(All lean cuts)	Chicken	(Most are fine,
Brisket	Cornish hen	but limit to an
Chuck	Pheasant	ounce per day)
• Chuck eye	Turkey	
• Pot roast		
• Short ribs	**Other Meat**	**Dairy**
• Top blade		
Flank	Game meats	(Avoid any that
• Flank steak	• Buffalo	contain trans
Ground beef	• Elk	fats, or added
Pastrami	• Ostrich	sugar or HFCS)
Plate	• Venison	Milk (skim, 1%,
• Short steak	• Yak	2%, or whole)
Rib	Lamb	Half-and-half
• Back ribs	Pork	Plain yogurt
• Rib eye	• Canadian bacon	
• Rib roast	• Ham	
Rounds	• Pork loin	
Round steak	• Pork tenderloin	
• Boneless rump roast	Soy-based meat	
• Bottom round roast	substitutes	
• Top round roast	Veal	
• Top round steak		
Short loin		
• Porterhouse		
• T-Bone		
• Tenderloin		
Sirloin		
• Sirloin		
• Top sirloin		
• Tri-Tip		

Table 7.4

Glycemic Index (GI)

Ranges of GI: Very low GI (10–30), Low GI (35–55),
Medium GI (60–69), High GI (70 and above)

Cereals		Breads		Vegetables	
Corn flakes	98	Bagel	72	Beets	69
Muesli	68	Blueberry muffin	59	Broccoli	10
Rice Krispies	100	Croissant	67	Cabbage	10
		Donut	76	Carrots	49
Grains		Pita bread	57	Corn	55
Brown rice	55	Pumpernickel	51	Green peas	48
Buckwheat	54	Rye bread	76	Lettuce	10
Bulgur	48	Sourdough	52	Mushrooms	10
Short grain		Stone ground whole		Onions	10
white rice	72	wheat	53	Parsnips	97
		White	70	Potato (baked)	93
Dairy				Potato (french fries)	75
Ice cream (low fat)	50	**Fruit**		Potato (instant,	
Ice cream (whole)	61	Apple	38	mashed)	86
Milk (whole)	22	Banana	55	Potato (new)	62
Milk (skimmed)	32	Cantaloupe	65	Pumpkin	75
Yogurt (low fat)	33	Cherries	22	Red peppers	10
		Grapefruit	25	Sweet potato	54
Cookies		Grapes	46		
Graham crackers	74	Kiwi	52	**Beans**	
Melba toast	70	Mango	55	Baked beans	48
Oatmeal cookies	55	Orange	44	Broad beans	79
Rice cakes	82	Papaya	58	Garbanzo beans	
Rice crackers	91	Pear	38	(chickpeas)	33
Soda crackers	74	Pineapple	66	Lentils	30
Stoned wheat thins	67	Plum	39	Lima beans	32
		Raisins	56	Navy beans	38
Pasta		Strawberries	42	Pinto beans	39
Capellini	45	Watermelon	103	Red kidney beans	27
Fettuccini	32			Soy beans	18
Linguini	46	**Sugars**		White beans	31
Macaroni	47	Fructose	23		
Rice vermicelli	58	Glucose	100	**Snack Foods**	
Spaghetti	43	Honey	58	Chocolate bar	49
Spiral pasta	43	Lactose	46	Corn chips	72
		Maltose	105	Jelly beans	80
		Sucrose		Popcorn	72
		(table sugar)	65	Pretzels	83

Table 7.5

Note that the GI has been criticized for the following reasons:

- It does not take into account other health-related factors (such as the insulin response) in the interpretation of the glycemic response to carbohydrates.

- The GI is significantly altered by the state of the food, such as ripeness, processing, storage, and cooking methods (baked potatoes versus mashed potatoes versus fried potatoes, for example).

- The GI varies from person to person.

- Sugars such as fructose have a low GI, but when used excessively (more than 4 grams per day), they are bad for your health for other reasons (such as contributing to the development of insulin resistance, diabetes, and obesity). The take-home message is that sugars should be avoided even though some of them have a low GI.

Since it is not practical to determine the GI for each food in all humans, the GI guidelines are a good indicator of how, on average, your body will react to various carbohydrate-containing foods. They should be used as a handy guide. To take a more sophisticated approach, one must be aware that the state of the food makes a difference in its GI. Mechanically treating the food (such as mashing potatoes) increases its GI. By pre-treating the food with heat (i.e., cooking it rather than eating it raw), the GI may increase. Similarly, riper foods tend to have a higher GI. In addition, certain sugars (fructose and HFCS) have a low GI rating but should be avoided for other reasons. With these caveats in mind, consulting the GI in table 7.5, and using it to assist you in making food choices, can be very helpful.

Benefits of Herbs and Spices

These tasty seasonings can add much more than flavor, color, and variety to your favorite foods. Every time you flavor your meals with herbs and spices you are literally making whatever you eat "better" without adding a single calorie. Here are some reasons why:

- They maximize nutrient density because they contain vitamins, minerals, and antioxidants.

- They make the diet more thermogenic, which means that you burn calories faster, by increasing your metabolism.

- Some even make you feel fuller. One study demonstrated that eating ½ teaspoon of red pepper flakes before a meal decreased subsequent calorie intake by 10 to 15 percent.

- The complex flavors they impart decrease the need for salt.

- Certain herbs and spices (such as cinnamon and coriander) allow your body to handle glucose more effectively.

- Others (cumin, sage, and turmeric) improve brain health.

- Basil, cinnamon, thyme, saffron, and ginger have immune-boosting powers.

- Many herbs and spices have distinctive health-promoting properties as well.

- Herbs can be used fresh or after they have been dried. Fresh herbs are tastier in salads. Dried herbs, when used in cooking, require time to absorb the oils, flavors, and other foods they are mixed with. Dried herbs tend to concentrate their nutrients, so smaller amounts are required. During the drying process some of the volatile oils and a small portion of the other components can be lost, but the overall nutritional profile is quite similar.

- Herbs and spices are concentrated sources of phytonutrients (plant nutrients), so it is not necessary to use large amounts. What is probably more important is to use combinations of herbs and spices in each dish. This enhances the resulting flavor and amplifies the synergistic benefits of the nutrients.

Brain-Belly Basics

Basil, cinnamon, thyme, saffron, and ginger have immune-boosting powers.

Here in detail are some of my favorite herbs and spices and what they "bring to the table," nutritionally speaking.

Herbs and Spices
(Use liberally, mix freely, and be creative!)

Allspice	Cinnamon	Oregano
Anise	Clove	Paprika
Basil	Coriander	Parsley
Bay leaf	Cumin	Pepper
Caraway	Dill	Poppy seed
Cardamom	Dill seed	Red pepper
Cayenne pepper	Fennel	Rosemary
Celery seed	Garlic	Saffron
Chervil	Ginger	Sage
Chicory	Horseradish	Thyme
Chili pepper	Mace	Turmeric
Chili powder	Marjoram	Vanilla
Chives	Mustard	Wasabi
Cilantro	Nutmeg	

Table 7.6

Ginger

The active ingredient in ginger is gingerol, a compound believed to relax blood vessels and relieve pain. One of its most well-known benefits is to ameliorate motion sickness, nausea, and vomiting. For these reasons, it is helpful to people suffering from the side effects of cancer chemotherapy.

It also is anti-inflammatory, which means it may be helpful in fending off heart disease and arthritis, and it is chock-full of antioxidants that are powerful free-radical fighters. Free radicals are damaging chemical compounds that are generated by our bodies each day. They can break down the delicate fats, proteins, and genetic material in our cells.

Ginger is often served with sushi. Fresh ginger root even makes a soothing ginger tea. Dried ground ginger is typically used in baking.

Cinnamon

People with diabetes should be particularly aware that cinnamon is a useful tool to help control blood sugar. A study reported in the 2004 issue of *Diabetes Care* found that this tasty spice acts to prevent the development of insulin resistance—a condition that contributes to the abnormal blood sugar swings so characteristic of diabetes. It also reduces cholesterol and triglyceride levels. A study in the *Journal of Nutrition* found that cinnamon is one of the best sources of disease-fighting antioxidants.

Cinnamon comes in sticks and as a powder. It can be used as a garnish, sprinkled on top of a bowl of oatmeal, grated over espresso drinks, and added to help flavor curries and vegetables.

Turmeric

Curcumin is the component that gives turmeric its bright yellow color. Its potent anti-inflammatory effect provides the likely source of turmeric's benefits in inflammatory bowel disorders, cancer, and Alzheimer's disease.

Turmeric powder has a warm, peppery flavor similar to ginger and orange. It is used in curries, egg salad, bean dishes, salad dressings, and sauces.

Sage

Sage also has antioxidant and anti-inflammatory properties. It seems to promote better brain function, as documented by a study in the June 2003 issue of *Pharmacological Biochemical Behavior* that found significantly enhanced recall in subjects who received sage oil compared to those who received a placebo product.

Its slightly sweet flavor makes it quite versatile. Sage can be added to soups, salad dressings, and sauces, or you can sprinkle it over vegetables.

Parsley

Parsley is a rich source of antioxidants and other heart-protective nutrients, including vitamin C and folic acid. Animal studies using parsley have shown that it can inhibit tumor formation and can neutralize carcinogens, including those found in cigarette smoke.

Fresh parsley is much more flavorful than the dried variety. It is used in salads, soups, and casseroles, and as a topping on fish and meat dishes. Try it as a breath freshener at the end of a meal, too!

Oregano

Oregano contains thymol and carvacrol—potent antibacterial compounds. It, too, is a powerful antioxidant and is rich in phytonutrients. On a per gram basis, fresh oregano has:

- forty-two times more antioxidant activity than apples
- twelve times more than oranges
- four times more than blueberries

Fresh or dried oregano can be added to Italian dishes, salad dressings, egg dishes, vegetables, and much more!

Brain-Belly Basics

The primary tenet of the Feed Your Brain Lose Your Belly diet is to include healthy fats and slow-release types of carbohydrates in a caloric ratio of greater than 2 to 1.

Much time has been devoted to providing you with the tools and insights to know why certain food choices are preferred. You have invested the time and effort to understand a universe of nutritional concepts. Now the fun part lies ahead—getting into the kitchen and seeing how this knowledge translates into a lifetime of tasty and healthy meals. Chapter 8 provides you with a week's worth of recipes, for three squares a day, to help you apply what you've learned and start eating right.

The Feed Your Brain Lose Your Belly diet is unique for a number of reasons, not the least of which is that it is easy to use whether you are an omnivore, a vegan, or anything in between. Those who wish to avoid animal products can merely increase the amount of beans, legumes, nuts, seeds, and oily fruits in their diet. I would suggest to this group that they also include a B12 supplement and possibly an algal-based DHA product.

The science lesson is now over. Let's head into the food lab!

The 12 Essential Components of the Feed Your Brain Lose Your Belly Diet

1. The primary tenet of the diet is to include healthy fats and slow-release types of carbohydrates in a caloric ratio of greater than 2 to 1.

2. Fish is brain food. It is also a key food source for fat loss. Have fish several times per week. Choose fatty, coldwater species such as trout, salmon, tuna, mackerel, herring, sardines, anchovies, and halibut.

3. Add lean protein from both animal and plant sources. Eggs are a wonderful source of protein and long-chain omega-3 fatty acids. Some are even supplemented with extra DHA.

4. Incorporate sources of the shorter-chain omega-3 fat α-linolenic acid, which occurs most abundantly in ground flax seeds and flax seed oil. It is also present in walnuts (or walnut oil), wheat germ, pumpkin seeds, spirulina, purslane, parsley, broccoli, kale, spinach, cabbage, dark green leafy vegetables, and Brussels sprouts.

5. Include veggies and some fruits in the diet. Choose non-starchy varieties and berries of all sorts.

6. Nuts and seeds typically contain monounsaturated fats (MUFAs) and are generally good sources of potassium and magnesium. They are calorie dense, so go lightly and choose from a variety, including almonds, pistachios, walnuts, pecans, and cashews. Sunflower, sesame, and pumpkin are my favorite seeds. They may be eaten plain or included in salads and casseroles.

7. Spice up your diet. Herbs and spices make almost anything taste better and are antioxidant powerhouses that are calorie free.

8. Blend color into the diet by selecting fruits and veggies in all hues of the rainbow. Be sure to mix and match because different colors provide different nutrients.

9. Add avocadoes. They are an excellent source of monounsaturated fat, protein, vitamins, and minerals. Have a slice with salad; add as a side dish with the main entrée; or eat as a snack with berries.

10. Don't forget coconut oil. It is the best cooking oil and is a great source of energy because of its high content of medium-chain triglycerides, which act as powerful appetite suppressants.

11. Green tea is a super beverage—so enjoy it! Drink it hot or cold. Drink water: it is the body's natural hydrator! Coffee and teas are great additions to the beverage repertoire as well.

12. Have a glass of wine, if you like!

8

SEVEN-DAY MEAL PLAN AND RECIPES

In this chapter you'll find a varied array of dishes that I have enjoyed over the years. As you read through the recipes, please remember two things: (1) the brain, which is made of fat, requires a continuous supply of healthy fatty nutrients in the diet for optimal functioning; and (2) during the low-fat eating experiments of the past thirty to forty years, obesity and diabetes have become commonplace. If eating less fat has contributed to this disastrous situation, eating more of the right type of fat should certainly help, as I have discussed repeatedly throughout this book.

All of the recipes in this chapter are provided as examples of meals that are included in this dietary lifestyle. These menus are to be used as guidelines and jumping-off points for the universe of potential food combinations that should be limited only by your imagination. They are typical examples of the types of meals the most successful volunteers in our weight-loss trial prepared. Just remember to be creative; use plenty of herbs and spices; add color to each dish; and explore foods you haven't tried before. Make eating a special time of the day—one you prepare for and one you truly enjoy!

Note: In all of the nutritional information I have provided, I have used the "effective" carb concept, which means subtracting the carbohydrates that are considered fiber (and are not absorbed) from the total carb content:

Effective Carbs = Total Carb Content - Fiber Carb Content

DAY 1 1933 calories (fat 1012, 52%; carb 478, 25%; protein 443, 23%)
Fat to carb ratio: 2.2:1

BREAKFAST 1

Calories 453 (Fat 113 cal, Carb 182 cal, Protein 158 cal)

Frozen Berry Smoothie (1 serving)

1 cup frozen berries (strawberries, blueberries, or mixed berries)
½ banana
1 cup water
½ cup ice
1 cup regular cottage cheese
½ cup 2% milk
1 tablespoon ground flax seeds

Place all ingredients in a blender. Blend until the mixture is smooth and creamy. Pour and enjoy. This is one of my favorites. You can use raspberries, blueberries, strawberries, blackberries, or substitute/mix in other berries.

LUNCH 1

Calories 515 (Fat 385 cal, Carb 71 cal, Protein 59 cal)

Nectarine Ginger Chicken Salad (4 servings)

3 nectarines (about 2.5 inches in diameter), sliced
2 skinless chicken breasts, cooked and thinly sliced
1 cup celery, thinly sliced
1 cup almonds, thinly sliced
¼ cup scallions, thinly sliced

Combine the ingredients in a salad bowl. Add the dressing and toss lightly. Serve immediately.

Dressing

1 cup mayonnaise
2 tablespoons white wine vinegar
1 tablespoon honey
½ teaspoon curry powder
½ teaspoon ground ginger
¼ teaspoon salt

Combine ingredients and mix thoroughly.

SNACK 1

Calories 339 (Fat 227 cal, Carb 77 cal, Protein 35 cal)

(1 serving)

1 Gala apple
1 cube sharp Cheddar cheese (1 inch on a side)
¼ cup walnut halves

DINNER 1

Calories 626 (Fat 287 cal, Carb 148 cal, Protein 191 cal)

Broiled Minty Tuna (1 serving)

1 tuna steak (1 inch thick; about 6 ounces)
½ tablespoon olive oil

¼ clove garlic, minced
¼ tablespoon soy sauce
4 leaves fresh mint, chopped rosemary to taste, lemon wedges

About 30 to 45 minutes before cooking, rub the tuna lightly with the olive oil and let stand. Mix the garlic, soy sauce, mint, and rosemary. Immediately prior to cooking, rub the seasonings into the tuna. Broil 2 minutes per side. Serve with lemon wedges on the side.

Broiled Asparagus Stalks (1 serving)

6 stalks fresh asparagus
1 teaspoon olive oil
1 teaspoon balsamic vinegar
salt and pepper to taste
cayenne pepper

Place the asparagus stalks on a baking sheet. Coat with a mixture of the olive oil and balsamic vinegar. Add salt and pepper and sprinkle very lightly with cayenne pepper. Broil for about 4 minutes.

Sautéed Yellow Squash with Gruyère Cheese (4 servings)

4 small yellow squash, thinly sliced
¼ cup butter
½ fresh sweet onion, thinly sliced
1 clove garlic, minced
2 tablespoons fresh tarragon, chopped
¼ cup fresh basil, chopped
2 ounces Gruyère cheese, thinly sliced
salt and pepper to taste

Melt the butter in a large sauté pan on fairly high heat. Coat the bottom of the pan evenly. Add the sliced squash and onions. Spread them out and cook them evenly, stirring frequently until very lightly browned at least on one side (about 2 minutes). Sprinkle with salt and pepper while cooking. About halfway through, add the garlic and herbs. Remove the pan from the heat and place the slices of cheese over the squash in a single layer. Let sit for a few minutes until just melted. Serve immediately.

Dessert: Cantaloupe with Cardamom (1 serving)

1 cup chilled cantaloupe balls
¼ teaspoon ground cardamom
½ teaspoon fresh lime juice
4 to 5 chocolate shavings

Mix the melon balls, lime juice, and cardamom. Serve in a glass dish with a mint leaf and chocolate.

DAY 2   1,918 calories (fat 1021, 53%; carb 573, 30%; protein 324, 17%)
Fat to carb ratio: 1.8:1

BREAKFAST 2

Calories 489 (Fat 274 cal, Carb 171 cal, Protein 44 cal)

Yogurt with Fruit and Nuts (1 serving)

1 cup plain yogurt
¼ cup raisins
½ ounce pecans, sliced
1 tablespoon flax seed oil
almond flavoring—drizzle to taste
ground cinnamon to taste

Mix yogurt, raisins, pecans, and flax seed oil together in a bowl. Drizzle with almond flavoring, sprinkle with cinnamon, and enjoy! This is a great breakfast that is well suited for the on-the-go lifestyle.

LUNCH 2

Calories 476 (Fat 253 cal, Carb 130 cal, Protein 93 cal)

Smoked Turkey Tortilla Wrap (1 serving)

1 whole wheat tortilla
3 slices smoked turkey breast
3 slices avocado

1 tablespoon sour cream
¼ cup shredded Swiss cheese
¼ cup salsa
oregano

Heat tortilla in a skillet over medium heat until lightly browned. Arrange turkey strips, avocado slices, sour cream, cheese, and salsa over tortilla. Sprinkle lightly with oregano. Roll and serve.

SNACK 2

Calories 345 (Fat 154 cal, Carb 161 cal, Protein 30 cal)

Trail Mix (1 serving)

pumpkin seeds, lightly toasted and salted (about 20 seeds)
¼ cup dried sweetened cranberries
¼ cup pistachios, toasted and shelled
10 dark chocolate bits

Mix together and enjoy!

DINNER 2

Calories 608 (Fat 340 cal, Carb 111 cal, Protein 157 cal)

Lamb Chop with Herbs (1 serving)

1 lamb chop
2 pats butter, melted
fresh rosemary, chopped
dill seed
garlic powder
sage
mint

Mix the butter, rosemary, dill seed, garlic, sage, and mint and brush on the lamb chop. Broil or grill to taste.

Sautéed Peppers (1 serving)

½ cup red and yellow bell peppers, chopped
1 teaspoon hazelnut oil
1 teaspoon fresh fennel, chopped

Mix the peppers in a skillet, cover with the hazelnut oil, and sauté. Sprinkle with fennel and serve immediately.

Spinach (1 serving)

1½ cups spinach
1 tablespoon olive oil
1 teaspoon sesame seeds, lightly toasted

Sauté the spinach very lightly in the oil. Top with the sesame seeds.

Dessert: Broiled Pineapple (1 serving)

1 wedge fresh pineapple
cinnamon to taste

Sprinkle pineapple with cinnamon and broil until lightly brown.

Brain-Belly Basics

Add lean protein from both animal and plant sources. Eggs are a wonderful source of protein and long-chain omega-3 fatty acids. Some are even supplemented with extra DHA.

DAY 3   1,793 calories (fat 997, 55%; carb 427, 24%; protein 369, 21%)
Fat to carb ratio: 2.3:1

BREAKFAST 3

Calories 556 (Fat 265 cal, Carb 131 cal, Protein 160 cal)

Southwestern Ham and Cheese Omelet (1 serving)

2 eggs
¼ cup 2% milk
butter for sautéeing
2 ounces ham or Canadian bacon (sliced)
1 ounce grated cheddar cheese
1 tablespoon salsa
1 slice sourdough toast with butter

Whip the eggs. Add the milk. While cooking them in the butter, add Canadian bacon and cheese. Top with salsa. Serve with buttered sourdough toast.

LUNCH 3

Calories 459 (Fat 268 cal, Carb 100 cal, Protein 91 cal)

Healthy Spinach Salad (1 serving)

1 ½ cups spinach
1 carrot, grated
1 tomato, sliced
1 mushroom, sliced
4 ounces turkey, diced
sunflower seeds (about 10)
raspberries (about 5)
⅛ cup walnuts, sliced
salt and pepper to taste

Toss together the spinach, carrot, tomato, mushroom, and turkey. Top with dressing (see below) and sprinkle with sunflower seeds, raspberries, walnuts, and salt and pepper.

Dressing (1 serving)

1 tablespoon olive oil
1 teaspoon white wine vinegar

¼ teaspoon freshly squeezed lemon juice

salt, pepper, celery seed, and paprika to taste

Mix the ingredients and shake well. Pour over the salad and serve immediately.

SNACK 3

Calories 223 (Fat 157 cal, Carb 31 cal, Protein 35 cal)

Crackers and Nut Butter (1 serving)

4 to 5 Blue Diamond Nut Thins crackers

peanut or almond butter

Spread crackers thinly with nut butter.

DINNER 3

Calories 555 (Fat 307 cal, Carb 165 cal, Protein 83 cal)

Garlic Shrimp with Parsley (6 servings)

1 ½ pounds medium shrimp, peeled and deveined

⅓ cup butter

4 medium cloves garlic, crushed and minced

⅓ cup fresh parsley, chopped

2 ½ tablespoons freshly squeezed lemon juice

salt to taste

In a large skillet, heat the butter over medium heat until it stops foaming (30 to 45 seconds). Add the shrimp and garlic and sauté, turning frequently until shrimp just turns pink (4 to 5 minutes). Add the parsley, lemon juice, and salt and stir well. Remove the pan from the heat and serve.

Brussels Sprouts with Hazelnuts (6 servings)

1 tablespoon butter

1 pound Brussels sprouts, trimmed and quartered

¼ cup hazelnuts, chopped

¼ teaspoon salt

freshly ground pepper to taste

3 tablespoons water

Preheat the oven to 450°F. Position the rack in the lower third of oven. Place the butter on a rimmed baking sheet and heat until melted. Remove sheet and place the Brussels sprouts and hazelnuts on it. Sprinkle with salt and pepper. Roast for about 7 minutes. Sprinkle with water, toss, and continue to roast until tender and lightly browned (about 8 minutes more).

Candied Butternut Squash (6 servings)

1 large butternut squash, quartered lengthwise, seeds removed
¼ cup melted butter
½ cup pecans, chopped
¼ teaspoon ground cinnamon

Scoop the seeds out of the squash. Arrange squash, cut side down, in a baking dish. Pour in water to a depth of 1 inch. Bake at 350°F until tender, 50 to 60 minutes. Cool, then peel. Cut into ½-inch slices, return to baking dish, and top with the butter. Sprinkle with pecans and cinnamon. Bake an additional 20 minutes until glazed.

Dessert: Blueberries (6 servings)

3 cups fresh blueberries
whipped cream
1 ½ teaspoons cognac

Top each serving with 1 teaspoon whipped cream and ¼ teaspoon cognac.

Brain-Belly Basics

Nuts and seeds typically contain monounsaturated fats and are generally good sources of potassium and magnesium. They are calorie dense, so go lightly and choose from a variety including almonds, pistachios, walnuts, pecans, and cashews. Sunflower, sesame, and pumpkin are my favorite seeds. They may be eaten plain or included in salads and casseroles.

DAY 4 | 1,889 calories (fat 1280, 68%; carb 400, 21%; protein 209, 11%)
Fat to carb ratio: 3.2:1

BREAKFAST 4

Calories 374 (Fat 223 cal, Carb 126 cal, Protein 25 cal)

Steel-Cut Coconut Oatmeal (1 serving)

¼ cup steel-cut oatmeal
1 tablespoon dried goji berries
1 tablespoon walnuts, quartered
1 tablespoon coconut oil
¼ teaspoon cinnamon

Place oats and goji berries in 1 cup of boiling water. Cook until smooth and let simmer for 10 minutes. Shortly before serving, add the coconut oil and remove from heat. Sprinkle with walnuts and cinnamon. Add some milk or half-and-half, if desired.

LUNCH 4

Calories 503 (Fat 324 cal, Carb 118 cal, Protein 61 cal)

Greek Salad with Genoa Salami (4 servings)

1 tablespoon flax oil
6 tablespoons olive oil
3 tablespoons white wine vinegar
1 teaspoon dried oregano
1 clove garlic, minced
6 cups romaine lettuce, chopped
1 can (15½ ounces) garbanzo beans, drained
1 red bell pepper, diced
1 red onion, thinly sliced
1 cup fresh fennel bulb, thinly sliced
½ cup crumbled feta cheese
2 ounces Genoa salami, cut in strips
¼ cup Kalamata olives, pitted and sliced

Whisk the oils, vinegar, oregano, and garlic in a small bowl. Combine lettuce, garbanzo beans, bell pepper, red onion, fennel, feta cheese, salami, and olives in a large bowl. Pour the dressing over the salad and toss. Place salad on platter and serve.

DINNER 4

Calories 1,012 (Fat 733 cal, Carb 156 cal, Protein 123 cal)

Macadamia Crusted Salmon (1 serving)

1 salmon steak (1 inch thick, 6 ounces)
⅛ teaspoon salt
⅛ teaspoon coarsely ground pepper
1 egg white
¼ cup macadamia nuts, finely chopped
½ tablespoon olive oil
1 pat butter
1 tablespoon fresh parsley, minced
½ teaspoon lemon juice

Sprinkle the fish with the salt and pepper. In a shallow bowl, whisk the egg white until frothy. Dip the fish in the egg white and gently pat the nut mixture into the fish. In a skillet, cook the fish in the olive oil over medium heat for 6 to 8 minutes on each side. Meanwhile, melt the butter and stir in the parsley and lemon juice. Drizzle over the fish and serve.

Curried Cabbage (1 serving)

1 ½ cups cabbage, sliced
1 ½ pats butter
⅛ teaspoon
mild curry powder
salt and pepper

Sauté the cabbage in the butter. Add the curry powder. Cover and cook until tender. Add salt and pepper to taste.

Sautéed Swiss Chard with Bacon (4 servings)

1 tablespoon olive oil
1 cup bacon, diced

2 cloves garlic, crushed
1 pinch crushed red pepper flakes
1 pound Swiss chard, stems and leaves separated
½ cup vegetable stock
salt to taste

Coat a large sauce pan lightly with the olive oil and add the bacon, garlic, and red pepper flakes. Bring to medium-high heat. When the garlic has turned light brown, remove and discard. At this point the bacon should be crispy. Add the Swiss chard stems and stock and cook until it is almost evaporated. Add the Swiss chard leaves and sauté until they are wilted. Season with salt and serve.

Dessert: Baked Vanilla Custard (1 serving)

1 cup 2% milk
1 tablespoon sugar
dash of salt
1 egg
1 egg white
½ teaspoon vanilla extract

Combine milk, sugar, salt, egg, egg white, and vanilla extract and mix thoroughly. Pour into a custard cup. Place in pan of warm water and bake at 300° for 1 hour.

Brain-Belly Basics

Incorporate sources of the shorter-chain omega-3 fat α-linolenic acid, which occurs most abundantly in ground flax seeds or flax seed oil. It is also present in walnuts (or walnut oil), wheat germ, pumpkin seeds, spirulina, purslane, parsley, broccoli, kale, spinach, cabbage, dark green leafy vegetables, and Brussels sprouts.

DAY 5   1,978 calories (fat 1105, 56%; carb 562, 28%; protein 311, 16%)
Fat to carb ratio: 2.0:1

BREAKFAST 5

Calories 431 (Fat 197 cal, Carb 153 cal, Protein 81 cal)

Country Breakfast (1 serving)

2 poached eggs with salt and pepper
2 pieces bacon
1 slice honeydew melon
1 slice rye toast
1 pat butter
1 tablespoon strawberry jam

LUNCH 5

Calories 521 (Fat 406 cal, Carb 19 cal, Protein 96 cal)

Zucchini Soup with Italian Sausage and Gouda Cheese (4 servings)

2 tablespoons olive oil
¾ pound sweet Italian sausage
1 red onion, thinly sliced
3 medium fennel bulbs, halved, cored, and thinly sliced
6 cups chicken stock
3 sprigs thyme
1 medium zucchini, thinly sliced
6 ounces Gouda cheese, finely shredded
salt and pepper to taste

Heat the olive oil in a saucepan. Add the sausage and cook over moderate heat until golden brown (about 10 minutes). Transfer to a plate. Add the onion to the saucepan and cook at moderate heat until slightly softened (about 4 minutes). Add the fennel, stock, and thyme and cook until the fennel is very tender (about

45 minutes). Add the zucchini; cover and simmer about 2 minutes. Discard the thyme. Purée in a blender and return to the saucepan. Thinly slice the sausage and add to the soup. Season with salt and pepper. Rewarm and then sprinkle with shredded cheese. Serve.

SNACK 5

Calories 424 (Fat 215 cal, Carb 116 cal, Protein 93 cal)

(1 serving)

2 ounces beef jerky
15 cashew nuts
4 dried apricots

DINNER 5

Calories 602 (Fat 287 cal, Carb 274 cal, Protein 41 cal)

Moroccan Dinner Stew (6 servings)

2 tablespoons olive oil
2 teaspoons butter
1 onion, coarsely chopped
2 cloves garlic, crushed (or more if you like)
2 teaspoons turmeric
2 teaspoons cumin seed
1 teaspoon dill seed
2 teaspoons coarsely ground black pepper
½ teaspoon crushed red pepper
1 pound ground beef
2 cans (10 ounces each) whole tomatoes with juice, coarsely chopped
8 cups low-sodium vegetable stock
½ teaspoon salt
2 cans (6 ounces each) garbanzo beans, drained
½ cup golden raisins
⅔ pound green beans, cut into 1-inch pieces
1 ⅓ zucchini, quartered lengthwise and cut into 2-inch pieces
⅔ eggplant, skin on, coarsely chopped

Heat the olive oil and butter in a large skillet. Add the onion and sauté for 3 minutes. Add the garlic, turmeric, cumin, dill, and black and red pepper, and sauté 3 more minutes.

In a separate skillet, brown the ground beef, drain the fat, and transfer to large slow cooker along with the tomatoes, vegetable stock, sautéed onion mixture, and salt. Cover and cook on high for one hour.

Add the garbanzo beans, raisins, green beans, zucchini, and eggplant. Turn the heat to low and continue cooking until the vegetables are tender, about 2 ½ more hours.

Dessert: Chilled Coconut Banana Mousse (6 servings)

6 ripe bananas
½ cup 2% milk
2 tablespoons coconut oil
big pinch ground nutmeg
½ teaspoon vanilla extract

Peel bananas; place in a heavy freezer bag and freeze for 6 hours. Remove and cut each into 6 slices. Place into a food processor with the milk, coconut oil, nutmeg, and vanilla extract. Process until creamy. Serve immediately.

DAY 6   2,052 calories (fat 823, 40%; carb 565, 28%; protein 664, 32%)
Fat to carb ratio: 1.5:1

BREAKFAST 6

Calories 487 (Fat 148 cal, Carb 171 cal, Protein 168 cal)

Smoked Salmon (lox) and Cream Cheese (1 serving)

4 ounces lox
1 ounce cream cheese
1 tablespoon 2% milk

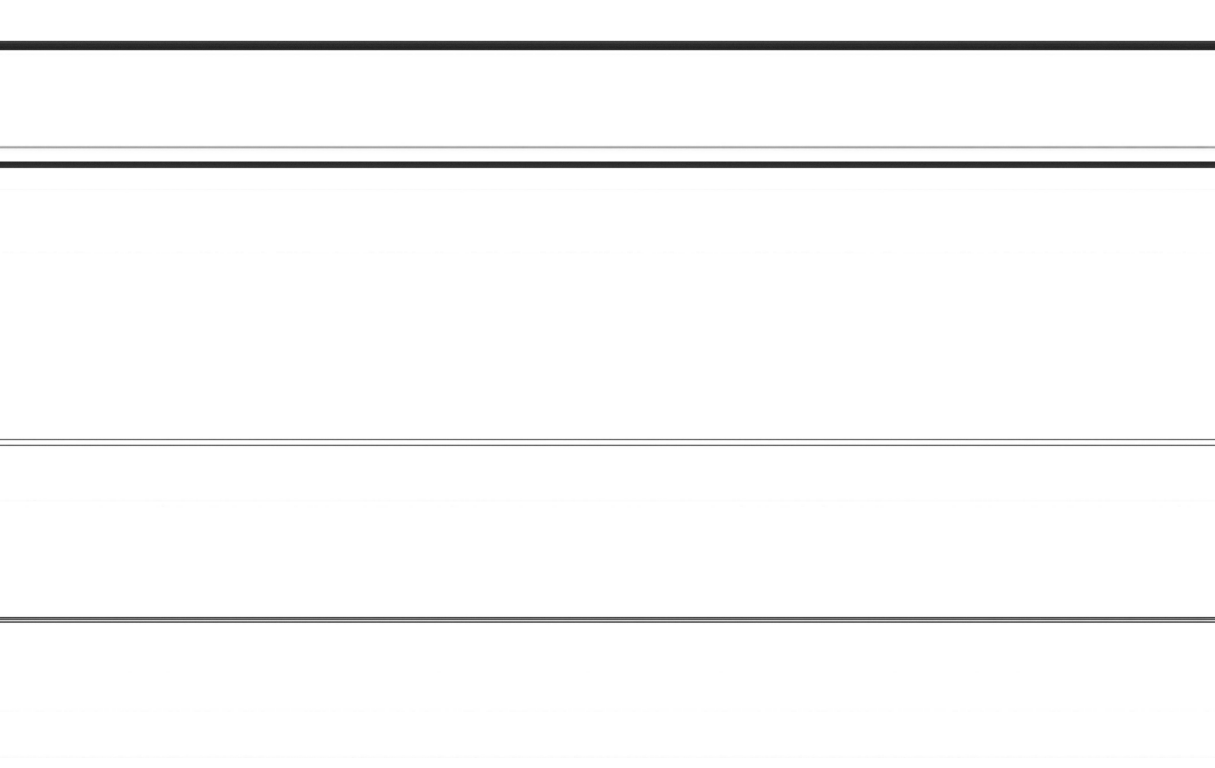

d this mixture on
nkle with several

n a large crisp leaf
and serve with dill

r. Add the buttermilk

(1 serving)

2 ounces provolone cheese

1 cup seedless green grapes

15 pistachio nuts

DINNER 6

Calories 702 (Fat 322 cal, Carb

Cranberry Orange

2 pork tenderloins (about 1 pou

2 large cloves garlic

½ teaspoon ground cumin

½ teaspoon thyme

½ teaspoon ground cinnamon

½ teaspoon ground allspice

pinch of ground cloves

1 tablespoon hazelnut oil

salt and pepper to taste

16 ounces fresh or frozen cranbe

1 can (12 ounces) mandarin oran

2 tablespoons sugar

juice and zest from 1 orange

Preheat the oven to 425ºF. Lightly

Mash the garlic and blend

cloves. Mix with the hazelnut oil

roast until the internal temperature

Meanwhile, in a saucepan co

and syrup, sugar, orange juice, an

mer for 8 to 10 minutes. Spoon so

cook for 5 more minutes.

Heat the remaining cranberry

pork stand for about 5 minutes befo

4 tomato slices
2 mini-bagels, sliced in half
capers

Combine the cream cheese and milk. Mix until smooth. Spread this mixture on the lox. Place atop a tomato slice on a half mini-bagel. Sprinkle with several capers.

LUNCH 6

Calories 470 (Fat 155 cal, Carb 86 cal, Protein 229 cal)

Grilled Chicken Lettuce Wraps (2 wraps = 1 serving)

4 ounces grilled chicken breast, sliced
1 cup tomato, diced
½ cup cucumber, diced
¼ cup carrot, shredded
2 ounces Buttermilk Dressing (see below)
2 leaves lettuce
2 dill pickles

Arrange the sliced chicken, tomato, cucumber, and carrot on a large crisp leaf of lettuce. Drizzle with the dressing. Wrap up burrito-style and serve with dill pickles.

Buttermilk Dressing

3 tablespoons sour cream
3 tablespoons mayonnaise
2 tablespoons white wine vinegar
¼ cup buttermilk
pepper to taste

In a bowl, whisk the sour cream, mayonnaise, and vinegar. Add the buttermilk and whisk. Season with pepper.

SNACK 6

Calories 393 (Fat 198 cal, Carb 121 cal, Protein 74 cal)

(1 serving)

2 ounces provolone cheese
1 cup seedless green grapes
15 pistachio nuts

DINNER 6

Calories 702 (Fat 322 cal, Carb 187 cal, Protein 193 cal)

Cranberry Orange Pork Tenderloin (6 servings)

2 pork tenderloins (about 1 pound each)
2 large cloves garlic
½ teaspoon ground cumin
½ teaspoon thyme
½ teaspoon ground cinnamon
½ teaspoon ground allspice
pinch of ground cloves
1 tablespoon hazelnut oil
salt and pepper to taste
16 ounces fresh or frozen cranberries
1 can (12 ounces) mandarin orange slices in syrup
2 tablespoons sugar
juice and zest from 1 orange

Preheat the oven to 425°F. Lightly oil a roasting pan. Trim excess fat off the pork.

Mash the garlic and blend with the cumin, thyme, cinnamon, allspice, and cloves. Mix with the hazelnut oil. Rub mixture over the pork. Place in oven and roast until the internal temperature is 155°F.

Meanwhile, in a saucepan combine the cranberries, mandarin orange slices and syrup, sugar, orange juice, and zest and bring to a boil. Reduce heat and simmer for 8 to 10 minutes. Spoon some of the cranberry mixture over the pork and cook for 5 more minutes.

Heat the remaining cranberry mixture to serve with the sliced pork. Let the pork stand for about 5 minutes before slicing.

Brain-Belly Basics

Don't forget coconut oil, which is the best cooking oil and a great source of energy because of its high content of medium-chain triglycerides (which also act as a powerful appetite suppressant).

Jicama Cole Slaw (6 servings)

1 head cabbage, shredded very thin
1 cup green peppers, julienned
2 carrots, shredded
1 Bermuda onion, minced
1 cup jicama, sliced

Jicama Dressing

2 teaspoons sugar
1 teaspoon celery seed
1 teaspoon salt
¼ teaspoon black pepper
1 teaspoon dry mustard
1 teaspoon cilantro, minced
1 teaspoon fresh parsley
¼ teaspoon ground basil
½ cup macadamia nut oil
1 cup white balsamic vinegar

Combine the cabbage, pepper, minced onion, and carrots. In a saucepan, combine all the dressing ingredients. Bring to a boil. Remove from the heat. While still hot, pour over the cabbage mixture, blending well. Cover and refrigerate for 8 hours or overnight. Add jicama and stir again just before serving.

Brussels Sprouts with Almonds and Pine Nuts (6 servings)

1 pound fresh Brussels sprouts

6 tablespoons butter
½ onion, chopped
salt and pepper to taste
1 tablespoon freshly squeezed lemon juice
¼ cup almonds, toasted and slivered
¼ cup pine nuts, toasted

Boil the Brussels sprouts in water until just tender, 3 to 4 minutes. Split one open to see if it is cooked in the center. Strain and place in ice water to preserve color. Cut into halves.

Sauté the onion in 2 to 3 tablespoons of the butter until translucent. Add the Brussels sprouts to the remaining butter. Cook over medium heat for several more minutes. Add salt and pepper. Don't overcook or the sprouts will become bitter.

Remove from heat. Toss in half of the almonds and all the pine nuts and lemon juice. Place in a serving dish. Garnish with the rest of the almonds.

Dessert: Chocolate and Raspberries (1 serving)

2 squares dark chocolate (1 inch on a side)
10 red raspberries

Brain-Belly Basics

Remember two things: (1) that the brain, which is made of fat, requires a continuous supply of healthy fatty nutrients in the diet to keep it functioning properly, and (2) that over the past thirty to forty years during the low-fat eating experiment, obesity and diabetes have become commonplace. If eating less fat has contributed to this disastrous situation, eating more of the right type of fat should certainly help.

DAY 7 | 2,037 calories (fat 981, 48%; carb 600, 30%; protein 456, 22%)
Fat to carb ratio: 1.6:1

BREAKFAST 7

Calories 488 (Fat 161 cal, Carb 135 cal, Protein 192 cal)

Simple Banana Almond Smoothie (1 serving)

¼ cup almonds
1 tablespoon flax oil
1 ripe banana
30 grams whey protein
1 cup soy milk
½ to 1 cup ice cubes

Mix all ingredients in a blender and blend well. Enjoy immediately!

LUNCH 7

Calories 431 (Fat 222 cal, Carb 142 cal, Protein 67 cal)

The Best Egg Salad Sandwich Ever! (4 servings)

6 large eggs
1 ½ tablespoons mayonnaise
salt and pepper to taste
¼ teaspoon lemon juice
½ bunch chives, chopped
2 celery ribs, washed and finely chopped
8 leaves romaine lettuce
8 slices whole grain toast

Creating the best egg salad sandwich requires properly boiling the egg. It must be boiled so that the center sets, yet stays moist. Then dunk the egg in a bowl of ice water immediately to stop the cooking.

Place the eggs in a pot and cover with cold water by ½ inch. Bring to a gentle boil. Turn off the heat, cover, and let sit for exactly 7 minutes. Have a big bowl of ice water ready when the eggs are done cooking and place them in the ice bath for 3 minutes to stop the cooking.

Crack and peel each egg and place in a mixing bowl. Add the mayonnaise and some salt and pepper and mash with a fork. Don't overdo it. Stir in the celery, lemon juice, and chives.

To assemble each sandwich, place the lettuce on a piece of toast, top with the egg salad mixture, and finish by covering with the second piece of lettuce and toast.

Enjoy with ⅓ avocado, sliced and a ripe plum.

DINNER 7

Calories 1,118 (Fat 598 cal, Carb 323 cal, Protein 197 cal)

Scallops with Endive (2 servings)

¼ cup extra-virgin olive oil
juice of 1 lemon
salt and pepper to taste
2 ounces almond oil
10 endive leaves
10 large scallops
1 tablespoon fresh chives, chopped
1 tablespoon tomatoes, finely diced

In a small mixing bowl, combine the olive oil, lemon juice, and salt and pepper. Whisk together to make the dressing. Set aside.

Heat a sauté pan and coat with the almond oil. Sauté the endive leaves until golden brown. Remove from the pan. Arrange 5 endive leaves on each plate in a star pattern.

Add the scallops to the pan and sauté until they are golden brown. Add salt and pepper. Remove from pan and place 4 in the center of each endive star. Place the fifth on top in the center. Drizzle 1½ tablespoons of the dressing over the scallops and along the leaves. Sprinkle the chopped chives and diced tomatoes over the leaves and serve immediately.

Spinach Mousse (4 servings)

1 pound fresh spinach

3 egg whites
⅛ teaspoon nutmeg
⅛ teaspoon salt
⅛ teaspoon pepper
2 ounces heavy cream

Blanche the spinach for 30 seconds, then dry thoroughly. Place in a blender with the egg whites, nutmeg, and salt and pepper. Blend for about a minute. Drizzle in the cream and continue blending. Chill for several hours until ready to serve.

Peppers with Orzo and Mint (6 servings)

1 can (28 ounces) Italian tomatoes
2 zucchini, grated
½ cup fresh mint leaves, chopped
½ cup grated romano cheese
¼ cup extra-virgin olive oil
3 cloves garlic, minced
1 teaspoon salt
1 teaspoon freshly ground black pepper
4 cups chicken broth
1 cup orzo
6 green peppers

Preheat the oven to 400°F. Pour the tomatoes into a large bowl and break apart. Add the zucchini, mint, olive oil, garlic, and salt and pepper. Stir together.

In a medium saucepan, bring the chicken broth to a boil over high heat. Add the orzo and cook for 4 minutes. Transfer the orzo to the large bowl with the tomato mixture. Transfer the chicken broth left behind to a 3-quart baking dish.

Slice the tops off the peppers and remove all the ribs and seeds. Place the peppers in the baking dish with the warm chicken broth. Spoon the orzo mixture into the peppers. Cover with foil and bake for 45 minutes. Remove the foil, sprinkle with the grated cheese, and bake until the cheese is golden brown (about 15 more minutes). Remove and transfer to a serving plate.

Brain-Belly Basics

Blend color into the diet by selecting fruits and veggies in all hues of the rainbow. Be sure to mix and match, because different colors provide different nutrients.

Dessert: Apricot Ambrosia (6 servings)

1 can (15 ounces) apricot halves, drained
1 tablespoon coconut oil
3 ounces sweetened condensed milk
2 ⅔ tablespoons lemon juice
4 ounces crushed pineapple
¼ cup slivered almonds
½ cup whipped cream
½ cup flaked coconut, toasted

Chop 6 apricot halves for a garnish. Set aside. In a blender, purée the remaining apricots and coconut oil.

In a large bowl, combine the condensed milk, lemon juice, pineapple, and puréed apricot mixture. Fold in the almonds and whipped cream.

In each individual serving dish, place 2 teaspoons toasted coconut and then ½ cup of the apricot mixture. Top with the apricot garnish and 2 teaspoons toasted coconut. Chill and serve cold.

The total nutritional information for the week (average per day) is

Calories–1,943

Fat–1,031 calories (54%)

Carb–515 calories (26%)

Protein–397 calories (20%)

Fat to carb ratio–2.0:1

My Favorite Snack

As a special treat, my favorite snack is my mother Heather's spicy mixed nuts recipe. I have these around to munch on when I get hungry.

SNACK

Calories 162 (Fat 120 cal, Carb 21 cal, Protein 21 cal)
Fat to carb ratio: 6:1

Heather's Spicy Mixed Nuts
(Serving size: 16 to 18 nuts)

1 egg white
1 tablespoon water
4 cups mixed nuts (equally divided between almonds, pecan halves, walnut halves)
2 tablespoons sugar
1 teaspoon salt
1 ½ teaspoon ground cumin
1 teaspoon paprika
¼ teaspoon ground ginger
2 teaspoons cinnamon
1 teaspoon nutmeg

Preheat oven to 300°F. In a mixing bowl, beat the egg white and water until frothy. Add the nuts and toss until well coated. Transfer to a wire mesh sieve and drain for 5 minutes.

Meanwhile, in a large plastic bag combine the sugar, salt, cumin, paprika, ginger, cinnamon, and nutmeg. Add the nuts and shake well to coat with the spices.

Spread evenly on an ungreased 15 × 10 × 1 inch baking pan. Bake until the nuts are toasted, stirring every 10 minutes (35 to 40 minutes).

Remove from the oven and transfer to a foil sheet.

How Many Calories Do You Need?

The caloric content provided by the meal plans listed above isn't appropriate for everyone. Again, it is merely illustrative because 1,943 calories a day may be too many or not enough for different individuals. I have included an equation below to help you determine an estimate of what your daily caloric requirements are.

The basal metabolic rate (BMR) is the number of calories your body consumes to keep you alive in the resting state, and it must be adjusted based on activity level. I have listed typical everyday activities to help you determine your physical activity ratio (PAR) for each day. To roughly approximate your total daily caloric requirement you must multiply the BMR by the PAR.

Total Caloric Requirement = BMR x PAR

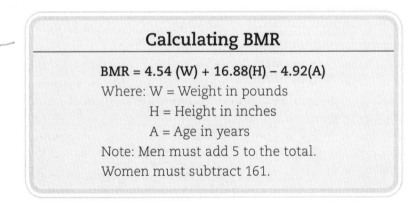

Calculating BMR

BMR = 4.54 (W) + 16.88(H) – 4.92(A)
Where: W = Weight in pounds
H = Height in inches
A = Age in years
Note: Men must add 5 to the total.
Women must subtract 161.

Table 8.1

Calculating PAR

PAR	Type of Activity
1.0–1.4	Sitting quietly, watching TV, writing, playing cards, listening to music
1.5–1.8	Sewing, driving, ironing, light office work, using the computer
1.9–2.4	Easy household chores, cooking, cleaning, dusting, washing
2.5–3.3	Dressing, showering, vacuuming, making beds, painting, operating tools
3.4–4.4	Mopping the floor, gardening, cleaning windows, moderate walking, playing golf, carpentry work
4.5–5.9	Chopping wood, brisk walking, dancing, moderate swimming, cycling, jogging, digging, shoveling
6.0–7.9	Very brisk walking, cross country skiing, stair climbing, moderate jogging or cycling, tennis, heavy swimming

Table 8.2

To calculate your average daily PAR you must determine how many hours of the day you do certain activities and assign each activity a PAR value. Then multiply the PAR value by the fraction of the day it is performed, and add them all up as shown below.

- Assume you sleep for 9 hours a day. (PAR = 1)
- You exercise vigorously for 1 hour a day. (PAR = 7)
- You perform light office work for 8 hours. (PAR = 1.7)
- You perform housework for 2 hours. (PAR = 2.1)

- You spend 1 hour showering, dressing, making the bed, etc. (PAR = 2.7)

- You do 2 hours of computer work at home. (PAR = 1.5)

- You watch TV for 1 hour. (PAR = 1.1)

These activities total 24 hours—a complete day. To determine your average PAR, calculate what fraction of the day (for example 1/24, 8/24 and so on) you do each activity and add them all up as follows: (9/24) x 1 + (1/24) x 7 + (8/24) x 1.7 + (2/24) x 2.1 + (1/24) x 2.7 + (2/24) x 1.5 + (1/24) x 1.1 = 1.69. So your average PAR over the course of the day (24 hours) is 1.69.

To calculate your total caloric requirement, multiply that number by your BMR. If you are a 50-year-old female who weighs 155 pounds and is 5'5" tall, your BMR is calculated as: (4.54 x 155) + (16.88 x 65) - (4.92 x 50) - 161 which turns out to be 1,394 calories. To calculate your total caloric requirement, multiply the BMR by your PAR and you arrive at 2,356 calories (1,394 x 1.69). If you had been more sedentary with a PAR of 1.4, your total energy requirement would have been just 1,952 calories. These calculations provide a very rough estimate of the total number of calories you would need to eat to remain weight stable. They also demonstrate what impact exercising has on your total energy requirement.

You are now an expert on nutrition, proper food choices, recipes, and how to calculate your caloric requirements. As we all know intuitively, the body needs to move to maintain strength, flexibility, and endurance. Sustained activity each day even contributes to a healthier brain. So the next step in your total makeover is to get you moving—and to do so safely. The way our Biggest Losers started the process, albeit somewhat hesitantly, is what you will learn next.

9

MOVE IT TO LOSE IT

Getting in touch with your body is especially important when you are trying to lose weight. Emotional eating must be distinguished from true hunger, and boredom from starvation. Subtle alterations in body composition develop and must be recognized. Even how you think about food can change. Being physically active enhances your ability to detect each of these changes.

We were born to move, to be active, and to challenge our bodies. For this reason it is necessary to incorporate into our daily lives activities that elevate heart rate, stretch our muscles, and produce all the beneficial hormonal changes that make losing weight much easier. All of these things are great for the brain and the body, and they just plain feel good once you get used to them! It is no surprise that being active on a regular basis is part of a healthy lifestyle. And to reap the benefits you don't have to be Michael Phelps. Setting aside the time and sticking to it are what really count. Remember the Nike slogan: "Just Do It"? After each session you will feel more energized than you did after the prior one. Although most of us can begin moving in a safe fashion, it is best to get a doctor's okay before starting any exercise program.

A Big Waste of Time?

To properly evaluate the benefits of the Feed Your Brain Lose Your Belly diet and activity program, we tested it in a group of volunteers. You will be hearing about the results in chapter 12. I refer to the subjects who lost weight on the program as our Biggest Losers. When they began the activity part of the program, several of them thought it was going to take a lot of time—time they didn't have to spare. Yet, by the end of the study, those who most ardently resisted the activity program became its staunchest supporters.

If you haven't done anything in a while to break a sweat, it can be surprising how winded you become just from walking up a flight of stairs. That's why it makes sense to start slowly, pace yourself, and be comfortable. Otherwise, you might get hurt. When this happens, any activity or exercise program comes to a screeching halt. So, it is better to be the tortoise rather than the hare in this situation, which also helps to ensure that you understand and feel good about your increased level of physical activity. Stressing this approach during the weekly meetings with our volunteers helped remove any anxiety about exercising.

Brain-Belly Basics

It makes sense to start slowly, pace yourself, and be comfortable. Otherwise, you might get hurt. When this happens, any activity or exercise program comes to a screeching halt.

Another recommendation we heard repeatedly was that to facilitate compliance, simplicity and convenience were of paramount importance. Still another suggestion was to choose a friend with whom to exercise (literally an "exercise buddy" to help keep you on the program), to compare notes and to just plain enjoy the experience. This will help keep you on track no matter what the weather is like. The mere sight of a pedometer on one of the study volunteers generated support from coworkers, friends, and relatives, which made it easier to stick with the program. It also created new friends and walking partners. These were welcome and unexpected perks of wearing that funny little box around wherever they went. It was like a "yellow badge of courage."

When approached in this manner, working out soon becomes something to look forward to. Believe it or not, you might even start to feel cheated if you miss a few sessions. It can even help with sleep difficulties—both falling asleep and being able to sleep through the night. You'll feel rejuvenated after you get your blood pumping. And stairs will gradually become less of a challenge.

It was for all these reasons that almost everyone felt that

including some physical activity in their daily schedule was vital. It also became a personal challenge, with all of the participants pushing themselves to surpass what they had accomplished the prior week. This was easy to measure because all were given pedometers to wear and graphed the number of steps they took every day. A few of our experts were startled to learn how far one can walk without going outdoors—even though getting fresh air was so stimulating.

Many of the volunteers for the weight loss study were *very* heavy and *very* out of shape. For them, the act of walking to the mailbox was difficult. For these reasons, and because we wished to avoid any injuries, the "program" they followed was quite different than what would be recommended for someone only fifteen or twenty pounds overweight. It was designed to get them moving comfortably and safely, to take the first steps to a healthier life. They know that was the plan, and joining the gym was the next step in the progression.

The exercise part of the Feed Your Brain Lose Your Belly diet and activity program includes three types of activity: walking, weight training, and balance and coordination. Walking should be performed three times a week—usually on Monday, Wednesday, and Friday—for 30 to 50 minutes. We recommended that study volunteers perform resistance training twice a week—usually on Tuesday and Thursday—for 20 to 30 minutes. They rotated exercising the three body areas sequentially as follows: (1) upper body strengthening, (2) trunk activity, and (3) lower body strengthening. We were not attempting to make people muscle bound; the goal was to include some "power" training (weight training) that augmented the aerobic benefits of walking. Weight training is also great for bone health. Approximately ten minutes of balance and agility activities were scheduled whenever time allowed, typically several times per week.

Just like they recorded all that they ate, volunteers documented every workout by detailing in a personal logbook what activity had been undertaken. This practice allowed each subject to track his or her progress. The study subjects were counseled to adhere to the activity program but to stay within their comfort zone. This approach was recommended for three reasons: to avoid injuries, to make it easier to stick with the program, and to keep it fun.

Brain-Belly Basics

Keep it Fun.

We suggested levels of activity that were "mild" to "moderate" because we wanted everyone to feel safe and to have a stable foundation from which to build. We were hoping they would achieve a sense of well-being, an improvement in cardiovascular fitness, and enhanced strength and balance—all without stimulating appetite excessively.

Keep It Simple—Walk

Walking was the preferred form of aerobic activity in the clinical study, and it doesn't require a pool, track, or treadmill. Plus, it starts as soon as you step out the front door, so no gym pass is necessary. The local shopping mall was also a favorite venue because it was enclosed, which assured protection from the elements. It provided a safe and well-lit place to walk while also being a great place for people watching. Since we attempted to make our activity program as user-friendly as possible, this was a perfect solution because it allowed everyone to participate and enjoy it.

What seemed to work best was walking three times a week on alternating days for 30 to 50 minutes. Each session included a ten-minute warm-up and a similar ten-minute cool-down period at the end. Almost everyone started at 30 minutes and slowly extended their time to 45 or 50 minutes. Please note that if you have other health problems or haven't exercised in a while, you may need to start more slowly. If so, don't be discouraged; you'll be surprised at how quickly you will be able to increase your exercise time as your body becomes accustomed to the exertion and as you start to lose weight.

The warm-up and cool-down periods consisted of slower intervals designed to get the blood pumping and make sure there were no injuries. The main exercise segment consisted of a period lasting 10 to 30 minutes depending on where people were in the program.

During this segment, the volunteers used one of three approaches. (1) Each time they walked they increased their speed slightly compared to what it had been during the prior session but never to exceed the threshold that made it uncomfortable to carry on a conversation with a walking partner. (2) Others used a different approach consisting of intervals of faster walking (for two to five minutes) alternating with slower intervals. (3) Another method employed (during an individual session) was walking at a slowly increasing rate in a crescendo fashion to a peak speed, followed by a decrescendo back down to the rate at which the person had started.

All of these approaches are fine. Using one method and then another is also acceptable. It is important to mix up any workout regimen to keep it lively. What we stressed was getting into the habit of being active through walking—preferably with a friend—and making it a part of the weekly routine. All study participants wore their pedometers and kept track of the number of steps they took during their walks. These were subsequently entered into their logbooks.

Keep It Simple—Train with Weights

The second component of the activity program involved light resistance training. Working out with weights was usually performed every Tuesday and Thursday around the home, which made it simple for everyone. Easily held household objects weighing up to 20 pounds were identified. They became the "weights" that were hoisted several times a week. Bags of coffee, cans of soup or soda, five-pound bags of flour, sacks of wild birdseed, and plastic one-gallon water containers were easy to locate. Gallon containers are particularly useful because the amount of liquid in them can easily be increased as muscle strength improves. What they weighed could easily be determined by putting them on a bathroom scale. Some items were held in one hand while others required a double-handed grip. Light weights were used initially.

As people became stronger, they progressed to somewhat heavier weights. No weights were necessary for some of the other muscle-building exercises. Upper body, trunk, and lower body workouts were alternated throughout the week. Weight training is an intense form of exercise. If you have never done anything like it, you might consider seeking help from a certified trainer or an experienced friend. As you become stronger, you will need to use slightly heavier weights.

At this point in your reading, it will be helpful to take a moment to go over some terminology that you might not be familiar with. Imagine that you are holding a can of soup in your right hand. A *repetition* (commonly called simply a *rep*) is the act of moving the can through a full range of motion of any particular joint, for example, the elbow. A group of repetitions performed sequentially, usually six to ten, is called a *set*. Usually two sets of any specified exercise were performed for each of three muscle groups. This simple approach takes about twenty minutes to complete.

Let's walk through a typical session.

Arm and Shoulder Exercises

Arm and shoulder exercises strengthen the biceps muscle, the deltoid muscle, and the triceps muscle.

The Biceps Muscle

The biceps is the muscle that bends the elbow joint in an upward manner. Its range of motion begins with the arm hanging in a resting position nearly straight down. A can of soup or something slightly heavier is held in the hand. Start bending the elbow up until your hand is near your ear. The motion ends here before being reversed—which means slowly lowering your arm until the elbow is almost straight again. Repeat this six to ten times; that is, complete a set of reps. The other arm is then put through the same group of movements. Perform two sets for each arm. This completes the workout for the biceps muscles.

Brain-Belly Basics

repetition (rep) = moving through a full range of motion of a joint

set = a group of repetitions, usually six to ten

The Deltoid Muscle

The deltoid is the muscle that moves the shoulder. When you place your hand on the shoulder, you are feeling the deltoid muscle. With your hand at your side using the same can you just used (keeping the arm straight), slowly raise the hand through an arc out to the side until it is parallel to the ground. You will have moved your hand through a 90-degree arc. Now slowly reverse this motion. That completes one rep. Repeat this movement six to ten times and stop. Perform the same exercises on the other arm. This completes one set. After you perform the second set you will have exercised two muscles.

The Triceps Muscle

The third muscle is the triceps muscle. It straightens (or extends) the elbow joint. For this exercise, you will need a heavier can, such as a large juice can. Grasp it in both hands and hold it over your head with your arms straight up. Now bend both elbows 90 degrees by lowering the can behind your head. Pause, then straighten your arms again over your head. This is one rep. Repeat six to ten times to complete one set of triceps exercises. After you are rested, repeat the set. This ends the upper body strength training session. It will take about twenty minutes to complete.

Leg Exercises

Leg exercises strengthen the calf muscle, the quadriceps muscle (also known as the "quad" or the thigh muscle), and the hamstring muscle.

The Calf Muscle

Grasp a plastic one-gallon water container in each hand. Start with them only half filled. In a comfortable standing position, start by rocking up onto your toes. Hold that for two seconds, then roll back down onto the soles of your feet. This constitutes one rep. Repeat six to ten times. Wait a minute or two, then do a second set.

The Quad Muscle

Lunges are a good way to build up strength in the quadriceps muscle. I would suggest not holding any weights the first several times you perform this exercise. Try to perform a series of lunges, first on the left side then the right. Start in a comfortable standing position with your feet side by side. While keeping your back upright, take one step forward. As you do, lower your pelvis until your front knee is bent almost 90 degrees. Hold this position for up to three seconds. Straighten up, take the next step, and repeat the maneuver on the other leg. Repeat six times. This constitutes one set. If you feel confident proceeding, try another set.

After you become comfortable with lunges performed in this manner, you are ready to try and carry hand weights. To get started, try using light weights in each hand—something the size of a can of soup might be best. Perform the lunges as you did previously, this time using the hand weights.

The Hamstring Muscle

Knee-flexion training exercises the hamstring muscles. A simple way to strengthen them is by sitting on the edge of a chair. Sit up straight with your feet on the ground and your heels touching the chair. Starting with one foot, press and hold your heel firmly against the front of the chair. Hold this position for four or five seconds, then relax. Repeat six to ten times with the same foot. Now perform the same series using the other foot. If you can comfortably repeat another set, do so. This completes the lower extremity strength training.

Trunk Exercises

Trunk training typically strengthens your side muscles, abdominal muscles, and back muscles. Start in a comfortable standing position with your feet about a foot apart, then place your hands out to your side. This is the neutral position for the three trunk exercises below. Start without using any weights. The weight of your body will act as the resistance. When you are ready, try holding light weights (two- to five-pounds) in each hand.

The Side Muscles

For the sides, slowly lower one shoulder laterally to about a 45-degree angle. Hold it for three seconds, then perform the same maneuver in the opposite direction. This constitutes one rep. Perform six to ten reps. Repeat the set.

The Abdominal Muscles

For the abdominal muscles, start upright in the neutral position. Then lean backward 20 to 30 degrees until you can feel your abdominal muscles tighten. Hold that position for three seconds then return to neutral. That is one rep. As above, repeat six to ten times. This is one set. After a brief rest, repeat the set. This completes the abdominal exercises.

The Back Muscles

Starting from the same neutral standing position described above, bend forward about 45 degrees. You will feel the muscles in your back tighten. Hold this position for three seconds, then slowly straighten up. This constitutes one rep. Perform six to ten reps. After a brief rest, repeat the set.

It is important to do all of the resistance exercises slowly to gain full advantage of the challenge presented by each motion. Doing them rapidly creates momentum that reduces the difficulty of each exercise. If it is too difficult to do an exercise slowly, lighten the weight until you become stronger and can increase it again. When you have become comfortable with these exercises, you can begin to include others. There are many websites and other exercise guides you can use to become more adept at weight training. I also suggest joining a gym and working with a qualified trainer.

Keep It Simple—Improve Balance and Coordination

The third component of the exercise program incorporates activities that improve balance and coordination. Examples include walking on irregular paths, jumping rope, playing ping-pong, and hopping first on one foot, then the other. Although these activities don't sound very difficult, all of our volunteers felt they were important. I believe they also help prevent injuries by improving balance skills. They can be practiced separately or performed while walking.

Positive Feedback

This approach to exercise and activity was enthusiastically supported by everyone. It made them all feel better both mentally and physically, helped them burn calories, and created an *esprit de corps* among the group. The recommendations were the same for each participant. However, they were personalized and adapted to accommodate various schedules and routines. Each of the volunteers felt that this was a fun and useful part of the program and enthusiastically suggested that you incorporate a similar version in your activity regimen. Much to their surprise, by the conclusion of the clinical trial, many of the participants had progressed sufficiently to take the next step and join a gym or recreation center for exposure to a greater variety of aerobic and resistance machines. An unexpected benefit of the "move it to lose it" program was the increased zest for life that was engendered. Hopefully you'll experience that as well!

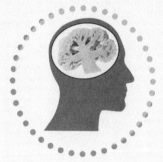

PART 3

You *Can* Train Your Brain to Lose Your Belly

10

DEALING WITH THE MIND-BODY CHALLENGES OF LOSING WEIGHT

Ten years ago, one in four Americans was obese. Now that number is one in three! On average, being obese usually means being about twenty-five pounds beyond just being overweight. Suppose you are a middle-aged female who is about 5'5" and your ideal weight is 125 pounds. If you weigh 150 pounds, you meet the criteria for being overweight. If you weigh 175 pounds, you are considered obese. About one-third (or more) of the weight of people who fall into this category is fat tissue.

This means they are carrying around almost sixty pounds of fat—upstairs, downstairs, while working, and even when exercising. No wonder it takes a toll on their bodies and joints. Imagine carrying a sixty-pound pack everywhere you go! If you were short of breath, it wouldn't be surprising. But that is exactly what many of us are doing. About 200 million Americans are overweight, and half of them (100 million) are obese.

Carrying excess weight is also associated with an array

of serious health issues, including diabetes, high blood pressure, stroke, heart attack, heart failure, certain types of cancer, gallstones, gout, osteoarthritis, and sleep apnea. As if those aren't frightening enough, we can now add memory loss and Alzheimer's disease to this daunting list. Needless to say, accumulation of body fat is a huge and growing problem!

In addition to taking a toll on us personally, the fiscal burden it imposes on the country's health-care budget is staggering. Annual health costs attributed to being overweight currently exceed $100 billion. This represents almost 10 percent of the total medical spending in this country. There are even current predictions suggesting that most Americans will be overweight within the next ten years!

With figures (and figures) like these, one might think there is something in the drinking water. Perhaps that is true. But there is definitely something in the food we eat. While genes clearly may predispose certain individuals to excessive energy storage (meaning fat storage), the emergence of widespread obesity has only recently become a problem. Surprisingly, not too long ago starvation was a much more pressing concern than obesity.

The Personal Toll of Being Overweight

Gaining significant weight usually takes a long time. It often requires months to reverse the process, if successful, and it isn't nearly as much fun. Large children get teased mercilessly. Adults fare no better. They feel the impact socially, professionally, and medically. It requires tremendous courage to embark on a weight-loss program. At this time, your friends, who should be your biggest advocates, often turn against you. (When you undertake a weight-loss program, it involves facing the fact that you are overweight. Many overweight people can't stand admitting it. When they see their overweight friend start exercising, this realization is sometimes more than they can bear. They react by avoiding the person altogether.) Pursuing such a challenging course can be demoralizing, and going it alone can often prove overwhelming.

To make matters worse, losing weight is usually not the only hardship that must be confronted. No one attempting such an arduous quest can be successful without addressing an array of emotional and psychological specters. Deb K, a confirmed yo-yo dieter, will attest to that wholeheartedly.

She first realized she was too heavy when she was a teenager. It was at about the same time that her complexion flared up. At first she was unsure whether the problem was due to stress, boys, or weight gain—or maybe a combination of all three. But weight was clearly a factor. She later became aware of the social impact of being heavy when she was ridiculed by her classmates and had trouble getting dates. As she gained more weight, she soon realized that finding clothes that fit and looked attractive was difficult, so she started wearing looser tops that hung out over her pants in a futile attempt to hide her excess pounds.

Later in life she began to have shortness of breath when she walked up more than one flight of stairs. She questioned her doctor about this. He explained that it was because she was carrying around fifty extra pounds and asked her to imagine how she would feel if she had to tote the equivalent of two heavy shopping bags wherever she went. That's when it dawned on her that being overweight could have potentially serious health ramifications. She was well aware that her dad, who had been quite heavy for a long time, had died of a heart attack. The other thing that really bothered her was that she found it impossible to do many things that she had been able to do previously, such as playing tennis and skiing. Her body was failing her!

In addition to the adverse health implications associated with being overweight, how you feel physically can have psychological overtones. Todd D and Marie L said the thing that bothered them the most was the way they felt in their clothes—like stuffed sausages. Several others hated the way their bodies seemed to jiggle when they walked—a perception they were painfully aware of. Each movement was an ominous indicator of these changes—an indicator that was apparent for everyone to see.

Occasionally, psychological stressors provide the perfect backdrop for gaining weight. Life is hard enough. Financial worries, caring for aging parents or difficult children, and a myriad of other challenges only make it more difficult. Such was the case for Katrina R, who grew up in an abusive family. It seemed like whatever she did was not quite good enough: her grades were inadequate, her sports performances were not up to par, her bed was never made right, and her closets were too messy. In other words, nothing she did was ever up to expectations. She doesn't remember ever receiving a compliment from her parents, and she subsequently (probably subconsciously) married a man who shared many of her father's traits.

For her, food was more a nutrient for the soul than for the body. It was a reward for what she achieved at work, a comfort for times when she didn't succeed, and punishment for not meeting her own goals. For as long as she could recall, she had considered herself to be an "emotional eater." She received gratification from food, because it was the only positive factor in her life. Unfortunately for her, it contributed to her yearly ten- to fifteen-pound weight gain—adding an unwieldy sixty-one pounds to her petite frame over five years. When she started the clinical trial and had to forego her comfort foods, she was worried about how she would cope without the safety net they provided.

Possibly the most poignant reminder of the impact of gaining weight is the realization of the associated health issues and the attendant fragility of life. The potential consequences of these insights made each and every volunteer in the study reflect upon the fact that they might not be there to take care of their aging parents or growing children. This single observation was the most prescient and motivating factor that kept them on the program. Grappling with one's mortality can be intimidating.

How you feel inside your body, the way you relate to people, and how you think about food are all issues that must be dealt with. So you will need to dig deep and be mentally and physically tough. You'll learn a lot about yourself as you proceed with the Feed Your Brain Lose Your Belly diet and activity program. One of the most important tasks you will confront is how you'll react to a new way of eating and a new way of living. Getting in touch with your body will be the first step that will need to be taken during the transformation—and a transformation it will be, because you'll be a different person at the end of the journey.

Get in Touch with Your Body

This phrase means different things to different people, but it is probably the most significant principle that those who stay thin have mastered. When you begin a new way of eating, what is most important is becoming aware of the vague, often unfamiliar signals your body will be generating; understanding what they are telling you; and knowing how to respond appropriately. If you want to be successful at losing weight, getting in touch with your body is essential!

A different activity profile, novel dietary recommendations, and alternative nutritional guidelines will combine to produce quite substantial metabolic alterations. Some may occur immediately, whereas others will become apparent only after several weeks. Your body may require some time to adapt to them. It is important to take a moment to understand what these are and how they can influence the way you feel and react. Heightened awareness will facilitate the entire process. Knowing what to look for makes it easier to discern subtle changes at an earlier stage and to *avoid misinterpreting them.*

To get started let's talk about several of the pathways that will be affected. For any weight-loss program to be successful, you must burn more fat than you store. When you gain weight, you are doing just the opposite—storing more fat than you are burning. To reverse this process, you must change the way your body works. As a result, novel signals will be produced that you may not have experienced previously. You must be aware of them and be able to determine what message they are sending.

Preventing the development of sticky fat cells is an example of one of these changes. Not misunderstanding the new signals your body will be generating is another. This is worth discussing in more detail, because it can derail any diet in a heartbeat. I think it is safe to say that no one is going to stick to a diet if they feel hungry all the time. However, there are certain signals your body will be producing that might be misconstrued as hunger if you're not aware of them. As was mentioned previously, a falling blood sugar level can generate a hunger response if the fall is far enough. As the sugar level decreases, the body will tap into its fat stores. If it is unable to access its internal energy stores, it will need to tap into its external energy supply, which means eating more. This response is due to the hunger signal that is generated by the brain.

If you are following the guidelines of the Feed Your Brain Lose Your Belly diet, as your sugar level falls, your fat cells will release fat for the body to burn. It will take over for glucose as a fuel source, there won't be an energy shortage, and you won't need to eat at that time. However, whether you end up needing to eat or you tap into your fat cells and don't get hungry, both scenarios begin with a falling blood sugar level. This blood sugar change makes the brain aware of the potential need for some form of nutrition in the future. For this reason, as you make the transition from sugar to fat burning, your body will sense the change, and you will become aware of it. However, it should not be interpreted as hunger, but merely as how the transition to the fat-burning state feels. It is a perception that should be viewed positively because it is how weight is lost, and it is a transition we should be making multiple times each day. If you are not aware of how it feels, it might easily be misconstrued as true hunger and will prompt an eating response. That is the last thing you want to do if losing weight is your goal. So, be cognizant of what to look for and don't end up thinking the transition to the fat-burning state is a hunger signal.

Brain-Belly Basics

If you want to be successful at losing weight, getting in touch with your body is essential!

As you have seen, to lose weight without being hungry requires successfully making the transition from using external calories (meaning the food we eat) to internal calories (the fat stored in our pantries). Once this occurs, we're home free, because many of us have enough fat to last for a very long time.

The most efficient ways to facilitate this transition are to choose foods that contain slow-release carb sources and to add brain-healthy fats to each meal. The slow-release carbs blunt the fall in sugar while the brain-healthy fats speed up fat burning. They work together to make the conversion from burning glucose to burning fat much easier.

Brain-Belly Basics

It is easy to misinterpret the sensation generated by the transition from glucose to fat burning as hunger.

On the Feed Your Brain Lose Your Belly diet, the transitions from one fuel to another are small and appetite is suppressed.

However, a subtle transition still occurs. For this reason, it is important to remember that such a diet can produce feelings that may be misinterpreted as early signs of hunger. However, they are not signs of starvation or lack of food, but merely reflect a transition in the fuel mixture from carbohydrate to fat.

This is why being in touch with your body and knowing how to interpret what you feel is critical—it helps differentiate a normal metabolic transition from other perceptions. Probably the most meaningful way to describe this subtle distinction is to characterize it like the difference between wanting to eat and needing to eat. With this perspective, it is possible to identify the physiological shift from the fat-storing to the fat-burning state—the condition associated with weight loss!

Nicole R summed it up nicely when she said, "I never felt hungry, because there was no need to be hungry!"

Now for the Hard Part—Dealing with the Emotions

Learning how your body is going to react when you start making better food choices and begin an exercise program allows you to be ideally poised to tackle all the emotional challenges you will be facing. The volunteers in our clinical study went through similar adversities and have provided compassionate perspectives that they found helpful.

If you look around, the first thing that should strike you is that you are not alone! No matter how out of shape, over-weight, or depressed you are about being too heavy, there are many others who are in worse shape and need to lose weight even more urgently than you do. You should also acknowledge that losing weight might not be easy for you. However, I suggest you keep in mind the fact that many people have walked in your shoes, and a number of them have achieved their goals! While success is a great motivator, there will be times when, regardless of what you do, you find yourself stuck on a dreaded weight-loss plateau. This produces many negative reactions including desperation, anxiety, depression, and fear of failure. To maintain your sanity at times like these it helps to accept the fact that you will be dealing with a multitude of raw emotions. Sometimes that is the most difficult thing to realize.

Brain-Belly Basics

To maintain your sanity it helps to accept the fact that you will be dealing with a multitude of raw emotions. Sometimes that is the most difficult thing to realize.

Self-Esteem Is Key—Don't Let Your Weight Define You as a Person!

A number of the study volunteers had issues regarding self-esteem. As a result, many of them shared the misguided belief that "I am not thin enough = I am not good enough." Ostensibly this makes no sense, yet it is ingrained in our culture. Consider how models, actresses, and other females in various ads are depicted. Whether they are advertising cars, cosmetics, beer, or cell phones, it seems that thinner is better. Because we live in an age when this type of information dominates TV, movies, magazines, and the Internet, we are all exposed both consciously and subconsciously to the association of a waif-like body with success, beauty, and power.

With this type of upbringing and subliminal messaging, it is not surprising that young girls (and boys as well) develop problems of self-esteem as they mature. As time goes by, additional life stressors such as finances, work, health, and family-related issues may conspire to cause one's body image to become increasingly difficult to contend with.

Maddie W was so troubled by how she reacted to her weight gain that she was prescribed an antidepressant. Incidentally, among their many other side effects, antidepressants can be associated with weight gain and, like all medications, should only be taken under a doctor's care. In Maddie's situation, her medication made it more difficult for her to lose weight. This contributed to losing her sense of self-worth and the downward spiral that ensued. Once this type of thing happens, reversing the process can be extremely difficult.

The good news for Maddie was that she had a great sense of humor and even did some stand-up comedy. That provided her with a sounding board for her emotions and allowed her to vent about her life, her circumstances, and how they made her feel. Luckily, at one of her shows she met a wonderfully supportive young man who convinced her that she was indeed a good person. This sincere gesture of support and honesty allowed her to start feeling much better about herself and what she could contribute to society. Once she realized that there was so much more to life than having a stick figure, she started feeling better about herself and became much more successful at meeting her weight-loss goals.

How it feels to be overweight is never good, but it seems to affect us all quite differently and produces various responses. It might even generate different feelings at different times in one's life, depending on the situation and history of past experiences. Trudy K referred to her weight gain as an indication of inadequacy. She said if she was unable to control what she put in her mouth, there was not much hope of successfully controlling anything else. It was as if gaining weight was a metaphor for many of the failures she had suffered over the years—a different manifestation of the same underlying pathology.

Determine What Is Important in Your Life

Concerns about her weight had plagued June D for a long time. Her friends were "on her case," and she was in a tizzy about what to do. She was finding it increasingly difficult to walk the eighteen holes of golf she played every Saturday without feeling somewhat winded. Bending over to do the yard work she loved so dearly was now a chore as well. Her knees had begun popping and had started aching over the past six months. Though she was only fifty years old, it seemed to her that her body was starting to give out.

Working in a bank where she spent most of the time at a desk didn't help the situation. Being a "professional" woman was all she ever wanted. And she was good at what she did. Whenever a problem arose, she was the "go-to girl" for a creative solution. Worried that she was even losing that talent, she started feeling overwhelmed. It seemed like a number of factors had coalesced to make her feel inept, inadequate, and intimidated. This was uncharted territory. People had always looked up to her and respected her opinion. She felt like she was losing control.

About that time she went to visit her daughter Randi, who sensed something was awry. After several attempts, June finally opened up and the two spoke frankly for a few hours. Randi was able to react in an objective manner to her mom's predicament. Following her sage advice, June decided to devote more attention to her own needs. She carved out periods during the week that were designated as "private time"—a particularly important practice that might apply to you, too, because so many people are busy giving to others that they don't take the necessary time to address their own needs. She even resumed her favorite childhood hobby of playing the piano, which helped to rejuvenate her. And she created some much needed distance between her private life and her professional life. This combined approach also made it much easier for June to focus on her weight-loss program, which was made more enjoyable and successful via a group effort with several of her friends who also wanted to lose weight.

Work at It, Don't Get Depressed, and Accept Help from Others

For a number of reasons, becoming a Big Loser is not an easy accomplishment. You must realize there are numerous ways to get to the finish line, many of which are not direct, predictable, or easy. Just when things are looking good, you might let up and even gain one or two pounds. This has happened to each of our experts, often more than once! Instead of fearing it, it is best to assume it will happen and learn to deal with it.

Part of successfully confronting a wrinkle in your plans is having the mental toughness to work through it. This is where your focus should be. The consensus of the group was that if you approach things this way, you won't get depressed or feel overwhelmed. Midway through the weight-loss study Natalie G gained a few pounds. At about that time her young daughter thought she had become pregnant. Working through this situation was almost too much for Natalie to bear. The stress was a real killer, and could have been a diet-breaker as well. Luckily for Natalie, it wasn't.

Brain-Belly Basics

Stress can be a real diet-breaker.

Marti B made these observations about stress and hunger. "Another thing that was very important to me was distinguishing between how it feels to be hungry and the false sense of hunger that can arise out of stress—a response that doesn't merit eating. That might be the most important thing I learned during the support group meetings. My friends were there to help me. Knowing I was not alone gave me the courage to continue." This shows the dramatic impact a good support system can provide.

You're almost there. Now that you understand all the mental and physical hardships involved and where the potential mine fields are in any weight-loss program, you're ready for a few practical tips to jump-start your new life!

PRACTICAL TIPS TO GET YOU GOING

As you get started, you will learn a lot about what makes you tick. Many changes may be necessary in order for you to succeed. Some relate to your attitudes about food and eating. Others involve decisions regarding what is really important and how to prioritize the areas of your life. All of the changes depend on whether you are willing to take responsibility for the decisions you make and whether you can commit to yourself.

There are also a number of more practical considerations that make losing weight easier. They might not be intuitive, but they were very helpful to the subjects who lost the most weight in the clinical trial. Here are a number of suggestions they incorporated into their routines.

Weight-Loss Gems

1. Use a Logbook

Each participant in the study was provided with a spiral notebook that was small enough to be easily portable, but large enough in which to record daily observations, including food consumption, activities, stressors, sleep duration and quality, frustrations, questions, and suggestions. Dietary choices and activity levels are pillars of any weight-loss program, and they were recorded assiduously. This diary was referred to as their logbook and was usually carried around in a purse, knapsack, or briefcase. It never left the side of each study volunteer.

When they initially enrolled in the study, many of the volunteers thought keeping a detailed record was a useless inconvenience. However, as the trial progressed, this perception changed dramatically. By the end they were all vocal supporters who praised the critical role the logbook had played in the success of the weight-loss process.

Although the participants personalized their logbooks and used them differently, each person recorded the key items that have been referred to in the program descriptions. On a daily basis they measured and listed the weights and amounts of everything they consumed. A typical entry, for example, might be:

Salmon—4 ounces

Asparagus stalks—6 with 1 pat of butter

Garden salad—1-1/2 cups

Oil and vinegar dressing with Italian seasoning—2 tsp.

Salt and pepper

Non-sweetened iced tea with 1 slice of lemon (12 ounces)

This level of detail is important in order for you to estimate the number of calories consumed or the fat-to-carb ratio. The logbook was also used to keep track of all activities. The subjects each wore pedometers that tallied the number of steps they took during the day as they went for walks, did chores around the house, ran up and down the stairs, or prepared meals. A similar approach was used for the resistance or weight-training portion of the activity regimen.

2. Prepare Food Beforehand

When you are really hungry, shopping for or preparing food doesn't make sense. That is when you are obsessing about what you can eat immediately. Invariably, in this scenario you are not going to make optimal food choices. You are more likely to select whatever can be wolfed down without preparation.

It is best to undertake food preparation when you have sufficient time to plan and prepare high-quality snacks and meals. You can mix and match nutrient-dense, low-calorie choices in a creative fashion. Make munchies that are easily transported to work or that you can comfortably eat in the car when you are doing errands. Save those that are more appropriately kept in the refrigerator for home-based snacking. That way sugar, refined carbohydrates, and trans fats may be minimized, and your waistline will thank you.

Donald N swore by this approach. It prevented him from "going off the edge" many times. When he was able to eat some small healthy snack and wait for fifteen minutes, he wouldn't get hungry for hours. He now refers to this as his "fifteen minute" rule. It was so effective that many of the Biggest Losers adopted it.

> ## Brain-Belly Basics
> It is best to prepare food when you have sufficient time to plan and prepare high-quality snacks and meals.

3. Eat When You Are Hungry and Never Allow Yourself to Get Too Hungry

Many of our experts detailed what they snacked on when they began to feel hungry. The choices were as varied as the participants. Sammy J was a true believer in the celery and peanut butter approach. Michelle T swore by beef jerky, saying, "It was chewy, tasty, and expanded in my stomach." Kat N liked carrying around a mixture of almonds and pumpkin seeds with a few dried cranberries thrown in. "They provided a slightly salty sweetness that I loved. I ate a handful and felt satisfied for hours! They traveled well and stayed fresh for a long time. My coworkers even started doing the same thing. Remarkably, it helped several of them lose ten pounds!"

Marti B found success another way. "After you have crossed the line from realizing you need to eat to the real hunger zone, it's very difficult not to overeat once you start. You go from hanging on by your fingertips to an eating free fall." She went on to say that one thing that really helped was forgoing alcohol. "I must admit that I like a glass or two of wine with dinner. However, I frequently found that when I had something to drink it was harder to moderate what I ate. I guess my inhibitions were diminished when they needed to be even more discriminating. Alcohol also has a lot of calories! So cutting it out of my diet entirely was very helpful for me."

4. Your Pedometer Will Become Your Friend

"When I first saw my pedometer, I had no clue how it worked. I couldn't even turn it on. Once I figured out how to use it, I soon realized how inactive I was. It taught me a lot. When I finally became used to having it on my belt, I quickly learned how many steps I could add during the course of the day," said Maude F.

This was a typical response from the study participants. "I never realized that little box could help me so much." And it did in several ways—not just by encouraging more steps per day (steps that could be added very easily while one was doing other necessary things without taking much additional time), but also by the curiosity and support it aroused in people who asked about it as they saw it being worn day after day. A number of participants' friends and coworkers even purchased one for themselves.

The fascinating thing that Trudy W noticed was that coworkers would ask, "How far have you walked today?" Or when she looked as if she was on her way to the snack machine, they would head her off and tell her she was doing so well losing weight that they didn't want her to take a step in the wrong direction. They actually became ardent supporters and saved her a number of times, reinforcing her will-power in the process.

5. Reading Labels Is Key!

"It's amazing what is hidden in foods to make them taste good. Who would have guessed they put high-fructose corn syrup in ketchup?" remarked Todd B. "What does that have to do with tomatoes?"

Dottie was shocked that "partially hydrogenated sunflower oil is how trans fats appear on food labels. I knew they were bad, and although I checked every label for them, I didn't know that's what they were called in the food business. I guess they do it that way to pull the wool over our eyes."

Brain-Belly Basics

You'll be surprised at how many seemingly "nonessential" ingredients you'll find in prepared foods.

Most of the participants said they really benefited from the label-reading exercise. Almost uniformly they reported they were stunned by the hidden amount of salt and sugar in the food they brought home from the grocery store. They were surprised at all the seemingly "nonessential" ingredients such as flavoring agents, colors, and stabilizers contained in the groceries that filled their shopping carts. Whether you believe artificial sweeteners are safe or not, you need to be aware of where they are lurking so you can make informed decisions about what you put in your mouth.

So remember the next time (and every time thereafter) you go shopping, READ THE LABELS!

6. A Treat Rather Than a Cheat

We are not on this planet very long. While some of us eat to live, most of us also live to eat. In real life we must determine how we organize our schedules, decide what to do, and choose how and what to eat. There are no food police looking over our shoulders. Nonetheless, we make many good decisions but also some that seem counterintuitive. Despite knowing what we should be eating, we often make different choices that might not appear to make sense. However, that is part of life, and a part that makes life worth living (the living to eat part)!

Jodie R had this perspective in mind when she remarked to the group, "I am calling this tiramisu a treat and not a cheat." What she meant by this was that she had built certain "indiscretions" into her eating approach so she didn't feel guilty when they occurred. She was well aware of what she was doing and made up for it by being scrupulous about what she ate both the day before and the day after. By treating herself for being "good," in her mind that dessert was not a cheat because it was planned for ahead of time. Other dietary choices were altered to appropriately incorporate the treat into her meal. So the best part was she didn't end up feeling guilty about what she had done.

7. Use a Scale to Monitor Portion Size

You may be surprised to learn that you're eating far larger portions than you realize. Initially, until you learn how to accurately estimate correct portion sizes, use measuring cups to dish out precisely two-thirds cup of carrots, one-quarter cup of almonds, or some other quantity of food, and buy a small scale to measure the weight of each piece of meat or fish.

Shelly N's initial response had been that these extra steps were a colossal waste of time. Her daily schedule was already overbooked, and she literally found herself arriving late wherever she went. So it made no sense to her to unnecessarily complicate life further.

That all changed, however, when she had to estimate an array of portion sizes in front of the other study participants. She soon found that her ability to "guesstimate" what comprised a half cup or a quarter pound was far from accurate. Not only was she frequently way off, she always overestimated, so her daily calorie intake was always about six to eight hundred calories more than she thought. This was a surprising yet very common finding among most of the study volunteers. This simple demonstration made Shelly a true believer in the utility of the food scale, especially once she learned that it required almost two hours of hard exercise to burn off all those extra calories she hadn't realized she was consuming. After using the measuring devices for four to six weeks, Shelly realized she could make much more realistic estimates of her portion sizes.

This insight accelerated her weight loss, and her renewed success made her even more motivated to stick with the program. She was not the only one to witness the power of such a simple intervention. What she found quite fascinating was both that she been eating 25 percent more calories than she had thought and that despite eventually eating less (after beginning to use her scale and measuring cups) she was not any hungrier.

8. Wine Is Permitted—Just Don't Overdo It!

Enjoy a glass of red or white wine with dinner. There is a correlation between light wine consumption and lower body weight. Wine contains healthy nutrients and makes most food taste better. However, I caution against excessive wine consumption because it isn't good for the brain, the heart, or the waist.

As you pursue the Feed Your Brain Lose Your Belly diet and activity program, compile your own weight-loss gems. That way, when you are queried about how you did it, you can easily pass along what worked for you!

12

CLINICAL TRIALS 101: HOW TO ARRIVE AT YOUR WEIGHT-LOSS GOAL FASTER

In most other books that talk about how to lose weight, the recommendations are made by people who have an opinion about what works. An opinion can be correct, incorrect, or somewhere in between. Promoters of many diets merely provide anecdotal evidence that their diet works—evidence based on reports of a few people using the diet: for example, Jane Smith followed this diet for two months and lost forty pounds!

Why is it crucial for you to know this? Because anecdotal results can be misleading for a number of reasons. With anecdotal evidence you don't know:

- how well the diet was followed
- whether the weight was lost because of the diet or other extraneous factors
- what side effects the diet caused

- what the likelihood is that you will lose weight based on how well other persons did
- what other weight-loss efforts they might have been making in addition to following the diet

If you're going to spend the time and effort to learn about and stick to a diet and exercise program, you certainly want it to make scientific sense, to be safe, and to provide exactly what is promised. How else can you be sure that your program will deliver?

Studies called clinical trials are conducted to test hypotheses. Hypotheses are basically guesstimates of what might be true: for example, that a certain drug can lower blood pressure. Clinical trials are precise tools that investigate treatment plans, drugs, or surgical procedures under controlled circumstances in human subjects who volunteer to be participants. When a study is done this way, the results can usually be applied to a broader audience—assuming the extended group closely resembles the participants in the study.

The clinical trial process should also be used when any dietary regimen or nutritional supplement formulation is being studied or compared to conventional recommendations. Why isn't this usually done?

For one reason, conducting clinical trials is tremendously expensive. For another, the most conclusive results are usually obtained when the subjects are in a hospital and have their meals prepared for them so that everyone follows exactly the same diet. A third reason is that clinical trials generally must be conducted for a long time, and not many people volunteer for such a program.

Given these constraints, in most weight-loss trials scientists try to do the best they can to gather meaningful information while study participants live at home and do their own shopping and food preparation. That is the approach we used to evaluate both the diet and the activity program described in this book, as well as the unique nutritional supplement that was tested.

Gaining weight usually occurs over a long time period. Losing weight is usually not much faster. So, anything that can speed up the process is a welcome addition to a weight-loss program. I developed the nutritional product Vita-Loss to help speed up weight loss. Although it is not a drug, it has been put through some of the testing that a drug goes through. It is designed to be used with the Feed Your Brain Lose Your Belly diet and activity program. To evaluate how well both the diet and the weight-loss product Vita-Loss work, they were tested in a human clinical trial.

Before we discuss the clinical trial, I will take a moment to go over some details about Vita-Loss. It includes a number of vitamins, herbs, and other nutrients designed to work together to *speed up metabolism* and *suppress appetite*. It has no caffeine or stimulants in it. A university-based clinical study—conducted in addition to the clinical trial described in this chapter—showed that even when *a single dose* was administered, it sped up the rate at which calories were burned.

Description of the Human Clinical Trial

Clinical trials are complicated programs. To help you understand exactly what all the parts are and how they fit together to accomplish their goal, I have broken them down into smaller components. We will delve into each in some detail, because it makes sense to see what each does. This understanding will also be helpful as you come across references to clinical trials in some of the popular magazines being sold today.

As a physician, when I make a medical recommendation to a patient, I require sound evidence to support my advice. It is usually based on clinical trials published in medical journals. Understanding this is so important, I have included a full appendix discussing in detail what goes on when a clinical trial is performed (see Appendix 1).

Our Study Design

A study design describes each part of a clinical trial in detail: the purpose of the trial; how subjects are chosen; the detailed steps outlining how the trial is to be performed at each step along the way; and how the results are to be analyzed.

Purpose

We wanted to do two things: (1) compare one diet and activity program with another (the Feed Your Brain Lose Your Belly diet and activity program was compared with a traditional diet and activity regimen used by the volunteers in the clinical study); and (2) see how adding the nutritional supplement Vita-Loss impacted the weight-loss effect of the Feed Your Brain Lose Your Belly diet and activity program. To answer these questions we needed three groups of subjects to participate in a double-blind, placebo-controlled clinical trial. These groups are referred to as the three "arms" of the study.

Description of the Feed Your Brain Lose Your Belly Groups

Group 1—Those enrolled in Group 1 ate what they felt was a healthy diet throughout the study and followed their own activity regimen, which involved approximately the same level of exertion as those of the other two groups. They received placebo (inactive) capsules, although they didn't know it until after the trial.

Group 2—Those in Group 2 also received placebo capsules that contained no active ingredients to promote weight loss. In addition, they were asked to follow a particular diet and exercise program, namely, the Feed Your Brain Lose Your Belly diet and activity program that included walking with a pedometer for about thirty to fifty minutes three times a week; doing twenty minutes of light resistance training for two days each week; and performing a few minutes of balance training each week.

Group 3—Those in Group 3 followed the same diet and exercise regimen as did the subjects in Group 2. The only difference between the two groups was that the subjects in Group 3 received the product Vita-Loss instead of a placebo.

You can see, then, that the only difference between Group 2 and Group 3 was that Group 2 took the placebo and Group 3 took Vita-Loss.

Group 1 ate and exercised as they usually did and took a placebo capsule. Thus, the only difference between Group 1 and Group 2 was their diet and exercise regimen because they both took the placebo product. (Note that during the study, neither the participants nor the people conducting the study knew whether they were taking the placebo or the nutritional supplement.) The difference between Group 1 and Group 3 was that Group 3 used the Feed Your Brain Lose Your Belly diet and activity program and took Vita-Loss instead of following the conventional diet and exercise program and taking a placebo—as Group 1 did. Therefore, any differences in outcome between Groups 1 and 3 must be attributed to the combined effects of the Feed Your Brain Lose Your Belly diet and activity program and the nutritional supplement Vita-Loss. Differences in outcome between Groups 2 and 3 could be attributed only to the fact that Group 3 subjects took Vita-Loss rather than the placebo product, which Group 2 was given.

Performance

What happened after the subjects enrolled in our study were randomized into one of the three groups? All were followed in an identical fashion: their weight, fat mass, lean mass, blood pressure, and heart rate were tested every other week, and they were questioned about appetite suppression. They were also evaluated for side effects. No adverse effects were noted in any group.

Everyone attended meetings during which questions were answered, dietary understanding was refined, and compliance was assessed. (Compliance means how strictly each subject followed the study guidelines.)

When clinical trials are performed, three things are very important:

Clinical Trial Terms You Should Know

The study design we used is called a prospective, double-blind, randomized, placebo-controlled human clinical trial—quite a mouthful! It is referred to as the "gold standard" of scientific research. It is more believable than other types of proof when determining whether a product or process works. That is why so much time and effort went into the design and implementation of our study protocol.

Prospective means the study is going forward in time. Subjects are chosen specifically to fit the study description and must follow the study regimen. Retrospective studies examine documentation that has been created in the past (i.e., looking at information that has already been gathered), before study descriptions have been written.

Double-blind means that neither the participants nor the study coordinators (staff conducting the study) know who is receiving placebo or active product. This helps maintain objectivity throughout the trial for everyone—all the subjects and the researchers, too.

Randomized refers to the fact that subjects are not preferentially placed in any specific group. They are randomly assigned to their respective group by a computer program.

Placebo-controlled means that the active medication or nutritional supplement looks identical to the inactive product (the placebo), and no one knows which is which (placebo or active product).

Breaking the code means finding out which participants were on placebo or active product for the results to be analyzed.

1. That the groups being compared are chosen randomly

2. That they have similar makeup

3. That neither the subjects nor the researchers know which subjects are receiving which drug

At the end of the six-week study period, final body measurements were taken so that they could be compared to the measurements taken at the beginning of the study (baseline measurements).

Analysis

After each volunteer completed the study program, all of the information collected during the clinical trial was entered into a computer program that analyzed the changes in the study parameters we were evaluating—such things as weight loss, fat loss, assessment of appetite suppression, and so forth. Then the results were compiled and tabulated.

Results

After all of the data were entered, the study code was broken so that researchers could find out who was in each of the three arms of the clinical trial and determine whether there were any significant differences in their outcomes. Averages for each group were calculated and compared. (Note: The details of this type of analysis can tax the brains of even the most mathematically gifted. Here we will present only the results of that analysis.)

In the following section, we will discuss the results attributable to the Feed Your Brain Lose Your Belly diet and activity program. We will be evaluating the effect of the weight-loss supplement Vita-Loss in the section thereafter. During the six-week trial period, subjects in Group 1 remained essentially weight-stable, losing on average 0.04 pounds (less than an ounce) in six weeks. Those on the Feed Your Brain Lose Your Belly diet and activity program lost, on average, 4.4 pounds in six weeks. This means the Feed Your Brain Lose Your Belly diet and activity program alone was responsible for an average weight loss of 4.36 (4.4–0.04) pounds over six weeks compared to the conventional diet followed by those subjects in Group 1. That amounts to 0.73 pounds (almost three-quarters of a pound) per week! These results were statistically significant (meaning that according to scientific standards, they were valid).

More importantly, calculations for fat loss over the six-week trial showed that the Group 1 subjects gained 0.35 pounds of fat while the Group 2 subjects lost an average of 4.3 pounds of fat. Thus, there was an average difference of 4.65 (4.30 + 0.35) pounds of fat loss in six weeks between Group 1 participants who gained and Group 2 participants who lost while following the Feed Your Brain Lose Your Belly diet.

The researchers also looked at the percentage of subjects in each group who lost more than five pounds of weight during the study and found that only 6 percent of the Group 1 subjects accomplished this, while 40 percent of the Group 2 subjects did.

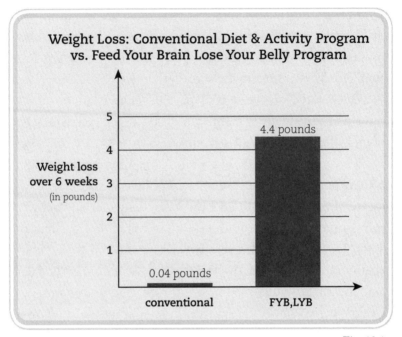

Fig. 12.1

The take-home message is that the Feed Your Brain Lose Your Belly diet and activity program was responsible for almost five pounds (4.65 pounds to be exact) of fat loss over the six-week course of the study.

We will now discuss the results of the nutritional supplement Vita-Loss.

You just read how successful the Feed Your Brain Lose Your Belly diet and activity program (when used alone) was at producing weight and fat loss. In this section we will discuss differences between the outcomes of Groups 1 and 3 and between Groups 2 and 3.

Group 2 vs. Group 3—The only difference between these groups is that the subjects in Group 3 were given Vita-Loss, so any differences in outcome between these groups are attributable to the nutritional product. As we saw previously, the subjects in Group 2 lost an average of 4.4 pounds over six weeks. The average weight loss for Group 3 was 11.77 pounds over six weeks—7.37 pounds more than Group 2—an average of an additional 1.23 pounds of weight loss per week. This weight loss can be attributed solely to the effects of Vita-Loss, because Groups 2 and 3 were on the same diet and activity program.

As you probably know, some diets have a greater effect on water weight loss than fat loss. If you've ever yo-yo dieted, I suspect you noticed how quickly your weight jumped back up if your loss was primarily water weight. So, your goal is likely to be to lose as much fat as possible. With that in mind, let's compare fat loss between the two groups. Group 2 subjects lost an average of 4.3 pounds of fat. Group 3 subjects lost 10.42 pounds of fat. This 6.12-pound difference (1.02 pounds per week difference) is attributable to Vita-Loss alone and demonstrates that 83 percent of the weight loss due to Vita-Loss was fat loss, not water loss.

It should also be noted that *all* the subjects in Group 3 lost weight during the trial! It is rare for all of the participants in any weight-loss trial to lose weight; generally, some of the volunteers remain stable or even gain weight during a study. These findings suggest, but do not prove, that most persons who follow the Feed Your Brain Lose Your Belly diet and activity program while taking Vita-Loss will lose weight.

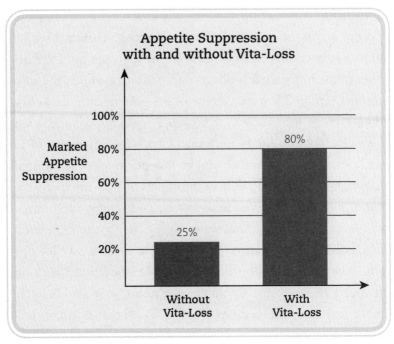

Fig. 12.2

All study subjects were asked about appetite suppression. By comparing the appetite suppression in Groups 2 and 3, we can determine how powerful an appetite suppressant Vita-Loss is. Of the volunteers enrolled in Group 2, 25 percent noted marked appetite suppression, as compared to an astounding 80 percent of those in Group 3. These findings demonstrate the substantial appetite-suppressing effect of the Feed Your Brain Lose Your Belly diet, which is greatly magnified by the use of Vita-Loss. The difference is statistically significant and is obviously of great importance for weight loss. Clearly, eating and food consumption increase caloric intake, so anything that

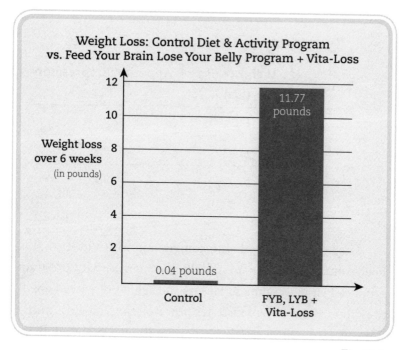

Fig. 12.3

decreases appetite should help curtail food consumption and speed weight loss.

Group 1 vs. Group 3—When Groups 1 and 3 are compared, the results reflect the combined benefits of the combination of the Feed Your Brain Lose Your Belly diet and activity program and Vita-Loss. Group 3 lost an average of 11.73 pounds (1.95 pounds per week) more than Group 1, and they had a fat loss of 10.77 pounds (1.80 pounds per week) more than Group 1. Most of the people in Group 3 also reported a marked reduction in appetite. It is also apparent from the analysis that 92 percent of the weight loss was actually fat loss, not water loss!

Summary of Clinical Trial Results

Group	Weight Loss (lbs)	Appetite Suppression (%)
1	0.04	0
2	4.40	25
3	11.77	80

Table. 12.1

The bottom line is that in conjunction with Vita-Loss, the Feed Your Brain Lose Your Belly diet and activity program produced large weight and fat loss and achieved marked appetite suppression. It demonstrates how well the Vita-Loss nutritional supplement and the Feed Your Brain Lose Your Belly diet and activity program work together.

The knowledge of how clinical trials are performed will help you not only accurately interpret results from weight-loss studies but also evaluate news briefs from magazines, the Internet, and newspaper articles. In other words, it will help you to see through the fluff, make sense of what is being presented, and separate real science from pseudoscience.

One of the things that keeps scientists honest, so to speak, is publishing the results of their research and clinical trials in peer-reviewed journals. Not all of the articles that are submitted are accepted for publication in these journals. Prior to publication, the articles are read by a review committee of unrelated scientists, who may be MDs, PhDs, or both, to determine whether each article merits publication based on both the quality of content and level of interest in the subject. The results of our clinical trial were published in a peer-reviewed medical journal called *The Internet Journal of Nutrition and Wellness*. The article (written by the person who performed the study, Dr. James Blum) was titled "Evaluation of a Combined Approach to Weight Loss." Although Vita-Loss is not mentioned by name, it was the product being studied.

This book was written for the lay public. With that in mind, I attempted to simplify complicated scientific concepts as much as possible. For medical professionals and any one interested in a more in-depth presentation of many of the scientific topics discussed in this book, a series of webinars is available at https://www.myimsonline.com/pages/Physician-Training-McCleary. This is the website for Innovative Metabolic Solutions—a group of dedicated medical professionals that provides content about diet, metabolism, and an array of health issues. The webinars qualify for Continuing Medical Education (CME) credit for doctors and other medical professionals and cost normal and customary fees for such material. People who wish to watch the webinars without obtaining CME credit may do so at a substantial discount.

To access the article, please go to: http://www.ispub.com/journal/the_internet_journal_of_nutrition_and_wellness/volume_7_number_1_21/article/evaluation_of_a_combined_approach_to_weight_loss.html.

If you would like more information about the weight-loss supplement Vita-Loss, please go to www.Vita-Loss.com.

APPENDIX 1

SCIENTIFIC RESEARCH APPLIED TO DIETARY SUPPLEMENTS

James M. Blum, PhD

Introduction

This guide is offered to those interested in the field of dietary supplement research and marketing. Reputable individuals involved in the research, production, and marketing of dietary supplements take research standards very seriously. First, there is the matter of formulating a supplement blend that is meant to benefit consumers in some way. Second, there is a rigorous and meticulous means of testing the product to determine if it actually has the intended effect. Finally, using published research data, supplement companies develop marketing strategies that promote the real benefit of their product to consumers who purchase it. The following orientation material is provided to aid non-scientific personnel in the understanding of the application of research to promote new products that benefit consumers and to support the reasoned and fact-based marketing of dietary supplements to consumers.

This guide is not meant to instruct lay persons how to conduct research. Only basic information is contained here. All dietary supplement research should be conducted by a credentialed investigator with experience in the type of research being conducted.

The terms *scientist* and *investigator* used in this document refer to the credentialed individual supervising or personally conducting the research study. Supplement companies are businesses who offer branded dietary supplements to consumers through sales.

Epidemiology Defined

We find that we cannot improve on the definition of epidemiology offered by Wikipedia:

> Epidemiology is the study of factors affecting the health and illness of populations, and serves as the foundation and logic of interventions made in the interest of public health and preventive medicine. It is considered a cornerstone methodology of public health research and is highly regarded in evidence-based medicine for identifying risk factors for disease and determining optimal treatment approaches to clinical practice (Wikipedia 2007).

Scientific Research

Scientific research is the study of scientific matters using what is called the scientific method. According to Merriam Webster's Online Dictionary, the scientific method is:

> the principles and procedures for the systematic pursuit of knowledge involving the recognition and formulation of a problem, the collection of data through observation and experiment, and the formulation and testing of hypotheses (Webster's Online Dictionary 2007).

Wikipedia presents a complete and concise expansion of the concept:

> Scientific method is a body of techniques for investigating phenomena and acquiring new knowledge, as well as for correcting and integrating previous knowledge. It is based on gathering observable, empirical, and measurable evidence subject to specific principles of reasoning, the collection of data through observation and experimentation, and the formulation and testing of hypotheses. Although procedures vary from one field of inquiry to another, identifiable features distinguish scientific inquiry from other methodologies of knowledge. Scientific researchers propose hypotheses as explanations of natural or artificial phenomena and design experimental studies that test these hypotheses

for accuracy. These steps must be repeatable in order to predict dependably any future results. Theories that encompass wider domains of inquiry may bind many hypotheses together in a coherent structure. This in turn may assist in the formation of new hypotheses, as well as in placing groups of hypotheses into a broader context of understanding. Among other facets shared by the various fields of inquiry is the conviction that the process must be objective to reduce a biased interpretation of the results. Another basic expectation is to document, archive, and share all data and methodology so it is available for careful scrutiny by other scientists, thereby allowing other researchers the opportunity to verify results by attempting to reproduce them. This also allows statistical measures of the reliability of these data to be established (Wikipedia 2007).

How Scientific Research Applies to Dietary Supplement Trials

Regulation

Federal laws under the purview of the United States Food and Drug Administration (FDA) govern medicine and dietary supplement testing on human subjects in the U.S. All human subject research conducted by universities, hospitals, or independent scientists must follow standards that are both comprehensive and complex. One of the many requirements aimed at ensuring safety and unbiased research results is that the study must be approved and overseen by an institutional review board (IRB). These independent boards are formed and commissioned by large medical facilities and universities. All scientific research using human subjects must have the sponsorship of an IRB. Boards vary in size but typically have ten to fifteen members—medical doctors, researchers, nursing professionals, university professors, etc.

A recent development that has greatly eliminated some duplicative administrative expense of numerous local boards is the development of the Central Institutional Review Board (CIRB) Initiative, sponsored by the National Cancer Institute (NCI) in consultation with the Department of Health and Human Services (DHHS) Office for Human Research Protections (OHRP). The CIRB provides an innovative approach to human subject protection through a "facilitated review" process that can streamline local IRB reviews of human subject research. This development eliminates the need for numerous local boards while ensuring study quality and ethics. Individuals who wish to conduct human subject trials must apply to an appropriate IRB and receive approval to proceed. All professional scientific investigators maintain a relationship with the CIRB or a local IRB in their area.

Human Subject Safety and Ethical Considerations

The principles of scientific research apply to every aspect of dietary supplement testing. From the scientific viewpoint, there is one important principle guiding supplement research to ensure the safe and ethical testing of products using human subjects. Medical research may involve laboratory studies using various materials and tools, animal subjects, or human subjects. The study of human subjects has historically been carefully regulated by the scientific community in the United States and around the world. Safeguarding human subjects involves:

- selecting people who do not have an underlying condition that might be worsened by the research

- ensuring that the product has no documented, historical ill effects to consumers

- ensuring that subjects have the capacity to provide informed consent

- ensuring that subjects indicate that consent via a signature

- carefully following the subjects during the course of the trial to ensure their health and safety

In summary, the study must ensure that the benefit to consumers is commensurate with or reasonable for any risk of negative effect that might result.

Efficacy

The practical goal of supplement testing is to determine whether the supplement actually achieves the intended or claimed results. For example, testing a weight-loss supplement will presumably indicate whether the supplement works in the manner intended; that it can be safely used in certain doses; and that study results are not due to coincidental matters. One characteristic of high-standard research is the use of control subjects. Using this method, a group with similar characteristics is selected and randomly assigned to receive a placebo (inactive look-alike product) or to receive the supplement being tested. This serves to remove the possibility of psychological factors affecting the results, because the subjects do not know whether they are getting the placebo or the supplement. Dietary supplement testing has been viewed with some skepticism by the medical industry and consumers because of a perceived lack of rigorous testing. Reputable supplement-research firms are dedicated to ensuring that the same testing procedures used in medical research are carefully applied to the study of dietary supplement research.

While this type of research requires time and resources, public safety and consumer interests require that supplement companies devote the time and money to quality research of supplements marketed to consumers.

Scientific Research Components

The following terms and phrases make up the common components of scientific research as applied to dietary supplements.

Acquisition of Subjects

The acquisition of appropriate subjects is a complex process balancing compliance with FDA regulations, IRB requirements, and the financial investment in a supplement that may not yet have gone to market. In addition, identifying subjects who meet the inclusion and exclusion criteria, considering the complex administrative logistics, is a combination of science and art. Acquiring subjects from among friends, employees, acquaintances, friends of employees, or other related scenarios clearly violates FDA guidelines and can put the study in jeopardy. Technically, this can lead to legal action against the owners, physicians associated with the product, marketers, and others associated with the product—it is *not* to be taken lightly.

Some investigators advertise for potential subjects using various media. This can bring study needs to a wide audience in a short period. Using this method, one can note the age and qualifying criteria and ask potential subjects to call for further information. Any method that identifies a random sample of individuals in a particular area may be used.

The process of handling potential subjects is outlined in the research protocol and follows FDA guidelines.

Adverse Events (ADE)

Adverse events are reportable to the IRB and to the company sponsoring the clinical trial. ADEs fall into two major categories: minor and serious. An example of a minor adverse event might be a one- or two-time belching after taking the assigned product. Examples of serious adverse events include gastrointestinal issues, rashes, vertigo, palpitations, abnormal laboratory values, and the like. The medical team makes a recommendation that the adverse event be identified as most likely not related to the trial, possibly related, or definitely related to the trial.

A common scenario is that an individual subject may experience a cold or twenty-four-hour flu during the trial. Initially, it may appear to be related, but if the symptoms abate quickly (24–36 hours) and do not reappear after additional dosages are consumed, it is generally deemed likely not to be related to the treatment. A rare event may include true cardiac disease such as palpitations or a myocardial infarction (heart attack), situations in which the results may be more difficult to categorize. Another less common scenario occurs when a subject receives a diagnosis of a serious illness such as cancer during the trial. Most serious diseases develop over a long period of time and are not due to the supplements under study. Professional investigators have a medical background that allows them to make recommendations to the IRB relative to any ADEs that occur.

Baseline Characteristics

In a study of two or more groups, analyzing the baseline characteristics is the most important method we can use to determine if the randomization of subjects into the various groups was unbiased or successful. Examples of baseline characteristics may include:

- age, height, and weight
- medical conditions such as
  –arthritis
  –asthma
  –depression
  –diabetes
  –gastrointestinal conditions
  –heart disease
  –thyroid deficiencies
- behavioral choices such as alcohol and tobacco use

If the vast majority of these characteristics show a similar distribution pattern between the groups, one concludes that the randomization was adequate and that no obvious bias is present. The interpretation of these analyses is somewhat delicate since even one or two unequal variables may present a challenge to the interpretation of a study. For example, in a diet- or weight-management study, if the placebo group had an unequal (higher) percentage of those with diabetes and thyroid disease, one may be concerned that the placebo group had a more difficult time losing weight independent of the treatment arm to which they were assigned. If, on the other hand, the treatment group had higher rates of these conditions and still lost more weight than the placebo group, it would indicate that the product might actually perform better in a larger population sample.

Baseline Testing

Baseline testing refers to the testing of subjects at the beginning of the study to establish a specific baseline measure with which the results or outcomes of the study will be compared. The baseline data are just as important as the final data points, and in some cases two sets of baseline data are obtained. This helps to determine whether subjects are too variable to be allowed to continue. For example, in a study based on laboratory values, if two baselines differ by more than 25 percent, the subject may be disqualified from entering the active phase of the study. This step helps ensure a higher chance of detecting a difference if one exists.

Biases

Bias can severely damage supplement research and the credibility of both the product and the company that sells it. It is the job of the qualified, ethical investigator to apply his or her training and expertise to identify and prevent bias from influencing a current study or to uncover overlooked bias that has influenced a past study. In the event of past study review, an investigator is retained to decide if bias has adversely influenced a given study, and if bias is found, to what extent. Wikipedia defines bias as a "prejudice in the sense for having a preference to one particular point of view or ideological perspective" (Wikipedia 2007). The most common form of bias identified in supplement research is that of a self-fulfilling prophecy in which subjective desire for a certain outcome drives the underlying aspects of the study. Consumers are naturally skeptical of companies that claim their product solves a problem previously thought to be difficult or requiring hard work by simply taking a pill.

One form of research bias is subject-selection bias, whereby subjects are inappropriately selected for the study. An example would be a diet study that does not exclude subjects with thyroid abnormalities. Since abnormal thyroid function could make losing weight easier or more difficult than for those without the condition, these subjects might bias the study.

This type of bias is prevented through careful development of inclusion and exclusion criteria and the consistent application of these criteria.

A systematic bias occurs when the study is flawed in its overall procedure, thereby resulting in a study that does not actually measure the desired factors. This is prevented by expert study design and implementation.

Interviewer bias is when an investigator conducts interviews that are influenced by his or her subjective judgments. This is prevented through training and research tools that minimize subjectivity.

Overt professional bias is at play when an unqualified or unscrupulous investigator designs a study biased toward achieving the desired result.

Confounding Variables

In epidemiological terms, a confounding variable is a variable that may influence study outcomes but may not have been acknowledged or accounted for in original research. In a study in which it appears that there are positive results due to the product studied, confounding variables can contaminate the study findings because they bring up other potential causes for the positive results (instead of the product that is being tested). Failure to treat confounders carefully or thoroughly may damage the interpretation of a study. An example might be a large national study of cholesterol-lowering drugs. Even if one controls for diet and consistent medication dosing, regional variations in the type and nature of food available in each area may affect the study result. Regional variations in the nature and type of foods available would be a confounding variable.

Being aware of potential confounders allows the investigator to control for them, thus making an "apples to apples" comparison possible. In the example of regional food quality, the investigator could isolate regions and study the data within each region.

Potential confounders are identified and accounted for in advance, as much as possible, during study design. Possible avenues for dealing with potential confounders include:

- control for potential confounders
- collecting data in a useful manner
- performing post-hoc analysis of these confounders

In studies with small sample sizes, assessing confounding variables becomes very difficult because of insufficient data to isolate data groupings and properly assess them.

Controls

Identifying the control group for a particular study is crucial for ensuring the usefulness and validity of study data. The ideal scenario is to use a true placebo, but some useful studies compare the efficacy of competitive products aimed at achieving the same consumer result.

The traditional choice is to use an inactive placebo to measure the background effect. This background effect is used to measure the net effect of the product. For example, in a weight-loss product study, if those using the active product lost seven pounds on average and the inactive placebo group lost three pounds, one would conclude that the real weight loss attributable to the product was seven minus three, or four pounds. The background effect is three pounds.

In other studies, the placebo group may actually move in the opposite direction from the product group, thereby enhancing the product effect. In a joint mobility product study, the product subjects may report an improvement of 20 degrees while the placebo group may report a 3-degree reduction in their range of motion. The resulting 23-degree difference may help the product group achieve a statistically significant result.

Dosing Instructions

Dosing instructions used in the trial should be simple and are supposed to be the same as those printed on the labels and boxes of the actual product sold in the marketplace. A seasoned investigator can provide advice about how to word these instructions during the development phase. Any differences between the label and study instructions may cause the results to come into question.

Dropouts

Dropouts are subjects who begin the active phase of the trial and do not complete all the requirements (visits or outcome measures). The most common and frustrating reasons for subject dropout are lack of compliance with the study or not coming to follow-up visits. Other, less common reasons include serious adverse events such as accidents, medical conditions, or illness. In the case of lack of compliance, investigators may be tempted to try to persuade subjects to continue, but the informed-consent requirements specify that human subject participation is voluntary—a subject is allowed to withdraw for no stated reason and may not be forced to continue against their will. The time, money, and energy required to screen each subject is considerable, and the research incentive is to have as many of the enrolled subjects as possible finish the trial. Sometimes a financial incentive is provided, but it is carefully monitored and subject to some debate by the IRB involved in each particular study.

An excessively high dropout rate may be considered a bias and subject the study to additional scientific scrutiny. As some studies are much more difficult than others, this is a vexing issue for both researchers and critics. A seasoned investigator must learn how to minimize this issue in his or her research.

Duration of Clinical Trial

The duration of the study is the duration (in days, weeks, or months) of the active phase of the trial. In weight-loss studies, the duration should be at least six weeks, although some experts prefer trials lasting ten to twelve weeks. Research tells us that most people can make and sustain dietary or lifestyle changes for two to three weeks before they tend to return to their normal habits. In order to reliably gauge whether a product related to these changes has a true effect, the active phase of a study must run longer than three weeks to compensate for this phenomenon.

Endpoints or Outcomes

The interchangeable terms *outcomes* or *endpoints* mean what is being measured. Examples include weight, lipid values, erectile function, sleep quality, and so forth.

It is generally agreed by experts that there should be only one main endpoint of the study with some secondary endpoints and safety endpoints included. Herbal or dietary supplement blends may affect a number of physiological systems and may seem appropriate for multiple outcomes. However, clinical trials maintain the highest validity and reliability when determining one primary outcome.

Using the optimal endpoint is a delicate balance that may involve medical equipment, laboratory testing, validated instrumentation, and financial commitment.

When designing a study, the question of which outcome is the most appropriate and how it should be measured is a crucial determination leading to trial success.

Exclusion and Inclusion Criteria

These criteria define who will and will not be enrolled in the study. It is essential to think through the medical aspects of every trial in advance to avoid undermining the chances of success. The purpose of the trial is to support scientific claims, and these criteria will define the data available at the end of the trial.

As an example, in a study involving an adult weight-loss product, who are most likely to lose weight? Women? Men? At what age? How does one deal with the fact that younger women may have an easier time losing weight but that product marketing may be directed to middle-age women? An experienced investigator will know how to focus the study to maximize the usefulness of data available at the end of the trial.

Subjects who give their informed consent are screened for the presence of criteria used to exclude them from the study. Exclusion criteria are designed to remove potential subjects from consideration for safety reasons or to eliminate the potential for other factors that may affect study outcomes. Candidates who meet the exclusion criteria do not go further in the study. The investigator screens each study candidate to ensure that the exclusion criteria are consistently and accurately applied. The development of exclusionary criteria is based on general safety concerns identified for particular medical conditions and the product being studied. A medical doctor may be retained to detect or confirm medical conditions. Samples might include subjects who:

- are unwilling or unable to comply with any aspect of the clinical trial protocol

- are allergic to or express problems with ingredients in the active product or placebo

- have severe co-morbid conditions (defined as any condition that would cause severe limitations or inability to carry out usual activities of daily living) including cardiac, pulmonary, renal, or hepatic disease or active cancer

- use prescription or non-prescription products that may affect the process being studied

- consume alcohol at an elevated level

- are insulin-dependent diabetics or have uncontrolled diabetes (as defined by A1c > 8)
- have had surgery or a hospitalization within the past three months
- have a cardiovascular event
- have an acute illness
- have a body mass index (BMI) of less than 25 or greater than 37.5 kg/m²
- have participated in a clinical trial in the past four weeks
- have any disease or condition that, in the investigator's opinion, compromises the integrity of the clinical trial or the safety of the subject
- women who are nursing, pregnant, or actively trying to become pregnant

Subjects who provide their informed consent are required to meet certain inclusion criteria specifically designed for the study. The investigator screens each study candidate to ensure the inclusionary criteria are consistently and accurately applied. Samples might include:

- women and men who are overweight or obese (BMI greater than 25 and less than 37.5 kg/m²) who wish to assess a beverage with the potential of assisting with appetite suppression and weight loss
- women and men who wish to promote healthy blood glucose management

- women and men who are eighteen to seventy years of age at the initial visit

Formulations

There are many ingredients on the market today. Determining the precise blend or formula that is to be tested is an art based on the science of what properties each ingredient has been shown to provide and how they may interact with each other. When testing blended supplements, the exact formulation used in the clinical trial must be the same that is sold in the marketplace.

Free-Living

In a weight-loss study, free-living refers to the instructions that subjects receive for a trial in which they are not placed on a specific diet or exercise program. They are asked to follow their normal diet and exercise patterns.

Hawthorne Effect

The term *Hawthorne Effect* was coined after a study involving industrial processing at the Hawthorne, Illinois, plant of AT&T's Western Electric Company. The Hawthorne Effect is when individuals in a study act differently simply because they are being observed. It can have such a powerful effect that techniques must be employed to ensure that it does not bias the study.

An example of the Hawthorne Effect can be seen in a diet study that requested subjects *not* to change their pre-study diet or exercise regimens. Individuals assigned to the placebo group may lose weight during the study simply due to conscious or subconscious seeds planted during a pre-study interview. As a result, study participants make slight changes in the type of food they eat, the quantities they ingest, and their level of physical activity. After detailed post-trial questioning following such a study with unexplained results, subjects will admit to making slight changes that affected the study outcome. A seasoned investigator is aware of this phenomenon and will take steps to minimize effects that can damage data usefulness.

Institutional Review Board (IRB) Approval

The primary role of an IRB is to protect subjects from unethical research. These boards work under Food and Drug Administration (FDA) guidelines and have circumscribed but strong powers.

An IRB works to protect the subject by assessing the research design using federal guidelines that cover such topics as the criteria for participation (both inclusionary and exclusionary criteria), laboratory testing, and other aspects of the research protocol. Additionally, they review the informed consent that potential subjects will sign in order to participate. Like all organizations, IRBs have preferences and areas of interest.

There are certain sections that they require and terminology they favor. Finally, their approval of all advertising and promotion (newspapers, radio, flyers, television, or Internet-based) is required.

The role of the institutional review board has grown in recent decades, but their origins go back to the human experimentation conducted by the Nazis during WWII and a few research projects in this country including the infamous Syphilis Trials. A summary of the issues involved in the American Syphilis Trials can be found in a *Science* magazine article: "Uses and Abuses of Tuskegee," by Amy L. Fairchild and Ronald Bayer, available at www.sciencemag.org (Fairchild and Bayer). Though we take subject safety for granted today, this was not the case years ago. The requirement that research be sponsored or approved by IRBs has greatly increased the safety and efficacy of dietary supplements and the benefits they claim to promote.

Seasoned investigator trials adhere to these requirements including, but not limited to, those listed below:

- The following FDA regulations should be incorporated into the conduct of research to assure that ethical standards will meet the worldwide rights of those subjects who participate in any study: FDA Regulations 21 CRF Parts 50.20, 50.23, 50.25, 50.27, 54.154.6, 56.107–56.115, 312.50, 312.52, 312.53, 312.55–312.62, 312.66, 312.68–312.70.

- Studies should be conducted in compliance with Institutional Review Board/ Independent Ethics Committee (IRB/IEC) informed consent regulations and ICH GCP guidelines.

- Studies should be conducted in compliance with all local regulatory requirements, in particular those which afford greater protection to the safety of the trial participants.

- All studies should be conducted according to the current revision of the Declaration of Helsinki (revised South Africa, 1996) and with local laws and regulations relevant to the use of new therapeutic agents in the country of conduct.

- Before initiating a trial, an investigator/institution should have a written and dated approval/favorable opinion from the IRB for the trial protocol and/or amendment(s), a written informed consent form, consent form updates, subject recruitment procedures (e.g., advertisements), and written information to be provided to subjects.

Informed Consent

An investigator must obtain informed consent from each subject enrolled in the study in accordance with the U.S. Food and Drug Administration (FDA) regulation 21 CFR Parts 50.20–50.27 and the laws and regulations of the country in which the investigation is being conducted.

The IRB must approve the informed-consent form and process to be used by the investigator. This includes ensuring that the subject has the legal and mental capacity to form intent and that they confirm their intent by signing a form. The investigator is responsible for ensuring that informed consent is obtained from the subject before any research activity is undertaken. This includes any diagnostic or therapeutic procedures as well as the administration of the initial dose of the study medication.

Matching Variables

One mechanism design experts use in minimizing potential study bias is to match study groups on certain variables. Specific variables will be controlled to be similar in both the treatment and control experimental groups. For example, by matching on sex (e.g., only women will be eligible), the groups are more similar. In a diet study, we might choose to have only female subjects in the study. The upside of including only females is that the population is more consistent, but the downside is that we cannot assess men with this study. Although this seems obvious in the case of gender, there are many other variables to consider that may not be as obvious or clear. Other matching variables might include age (within five years), BMI, or the presence of certain medical conditions.

Pharmaceutical-Level Clinical Trials

Describing a trial as pharmaceutical-level means that it meets the higher-order gold-standard criteria applied to the pharmaceutical industry. There are significant differences between non-pharmaceutical and pharmaceutical-level trials, including some or all of the following parameters:

- appropriate design expertise
- appropriate controls
- IRB approval

- sample sizes
- attention to potential biases (selection, Hawthorne Effect, misclassification, and others)
- endpoints
- laboratory work
- independent scientific oversight
- subject reimbursement
- duration of the study
- lack of a run-in period
- lack of various medical professionals (physicians, nurses, dietitians, respiratory therapists, etc.)
- lack of independent biostatisticians for the analysis phase
- lack of sophisticated medical measurement equipment

Placebo

A placebo is a product that looks identical to the actual product being tested but contains none of the active ingredients. The placebo must simulate the actual product in appearance while delivering a non-physiological effect. It must look, taste, and otherwise appear as if it could actually be the real product. It may *not* be a capsule with ingredients that couldn't pass the "straight-face test." If the real product is a blend of many different herbs and vitamin ingredients, one would expect a multi-colored and multi-textured placebo. It must be made so that a subject couldn't discern if they took it apart if it were the product or the placebo. The manufacturing of reasonable placebo samples may require an experienced manufacturer and may add a level of complexity.

Placebo-Controlled

The term placebo-controlled refers to the type of study in which a placebo group is compared to a group receiving the actual product.

Novices often wonder why a placebo or control group is necessary given that it drives up the cost of the study and may seem to diminish the effect of the product. However, in certain studies failure to use a valid control group (that is on a placebo) will mean that the results of the study are less valid and will be questioned.

A study that does *not* use a control is called an open-label study, defined by the fact that the subjects and staff *know* that they are taking the product. This type of study is appropriate in some situations. (See the section "Study Design Types.")

In a weight-loss study, the weight loss experienced by the placebo group should be subtracted from the product group. If the average weight loss in the placebo group was three pounds and the weight loss in the product group was nine pounds for the same period, then the actual weight loss due to the product would be six pounds. Without the control or placebo group, one might inappropriately conclude that the product was responsible for an average weight loss of the full nine pounds. When offering this product to consumers, an expectation of nine pounds of average weight loss is unrealistic and could lead to adverse consumer claims. Controls are employed to ensure we are measuring the true effect of the product. Without the control, the nine pounds is merely an estimate. There are times when the placebo group performs worse, making the actual effect that much stronger. In a study of an antiaging product using seventy-year-old men, several endpoints in the placebo group were reported as less-improved or weaker over the course of four months. The product group reported improved numbers over baseline, strengthening the effect of the product and helping make the product results statistically significant.

Randomization

Randomization describes the way in which subjects are assigned to the treatment/product group or control (placebo or other type of control) group. In a randomized study, neither subjects nor staff conducting the study know which group subjects are in, *and* each subject has an equal chance of ending up in either group. Study experts use randomization as a time-tested method to ensure that the results are valid. Since neither subjects nor the staff know the group assignment, subject responses are more likely to be their true responses.

Precise randomization methodologies are employed using "blocks." In studies involving two groups (product and placebo), blocks of six or eight are typically used. From every six subjects, equal numbers will be assigned to both groups. In this manner the overall numbers of the two groups will always be similar. In studies involving three groups, such as two products and a placebo, a block size involves a multiple of three such as nine or twelve. Standard randomization charts are used to determine the assignments, ensuring that all subjects have an equal chance of being assigned to the various groups.

Run-in Period

Run-in periods are short time frames at the beginning of a study used to establish baselines and test the compliance of new subjects. Run-in periods are typically one to two weeks in duration, but sometimes last longer when it is critical to develop laboratory baselines. They are useful for establishing more precise baselines and to weed out noncompliant subjects. The downside is that they increase the cost of a study.

Sample Size

The sample size refers to the number of subjects required to complete a study in order to reasonably expect to be able to document an existing difference. These numbers are derived from statistical calculations made during the design phase and involve a number of assumptions. They include such variables as the expected level of the primary outcome achieved by both the treatment and placebo groups and the chance of detecting a difference if one exists. Entire chapters of advanced statistical theory have been devoted to these issues. Readers who wish to explore these and other statistical topics should consult a technical resource or a reputable research firm.

Statistical Significance

Statistical significance is typically established at 0.05. This means that the differences one observes between the placebo and product results have a 5 percent chance of occurring randomly. It is thought that a one in twenty chance virtually assures that the results (if different) are "real" and not due to chance alone.

Study Design Types

The study design is a blueprint that defines the study structure. It provides all the basic principles and parameters and defines research strategies. An investigator must make informed choices in putting a study together. There are three major study structures:

Parallel Group: In this study there are two or more groups where subjects are randomized to one of the groups and are followed for the duration of the study.

Crossover: In this design, subjects start in one group (product or placebo/control) and are followed for a specified time period. At a set point, there is a short washout period during which they don't take any product, and then switch over to the other group (if they start on product, they switch to placebo, or vice versa). In this case, each subject acts as his or her own control. The advantage of this approach is that fewer subjects are needed to achieve statistical significance. The disadvantage is that the study takes more than twice as long to complete. The costs are about the same, but some product categories are better for crossover designs.

Open-Label: In an open-label trial, both the subjects and staff know that they are taking product, and no placebo or control is involved.

Subject Compensation

Compensation is an amount in dollars paid to subjects who complete the trial. Typically in dietary supplement trials subjects receive between $100 and $200 based on the trial difficulty and duration. Even at $100, if the trial involves sixty subjects to complete, this is a $6,000 budgetary item.

The amount and terms of the compensation are determined by the IRB involved in the trial. In cases involving partial completion, some IRBs require payment per visit regardless of the usefulness of the data obtained. This is particularly onerous because money is spent on data that may not end up contributing to study outcomes.

Types of Studies or Trials

Marketing Studies

The purpose of a marketing study generally includes soft endpoints which involve subjective criteria (taste, texture, appeal) rather than actual efficacy-type endpoints (blood levels, weight loss, etc.) that may involve some of the following parameters. Examples of soft endpoints are:

- taste
- texture
- aroma

- sensation
- usefulness
- delivery system
- efficacy

Marketing studies may be conducted once clinical trial research has confirmed a particular endpoint to aid in positioning the product with consumers or to refine a marketing campaign that has fallen short of plans and goals. These studies are not required to meet industry standards for human-subject research.

Pilot Clinical Trials (Proof-of-Concept)

A pilot trial is the same as a full trial except that it differs in the sample size. A pilot trial may be completed with only a quarter or a third of the numbers required to demonstrate statistical significance in a full trial. Companies often begin the process by ordering a pilot trial in order to conserve funds and to increase the chance of generating useful data in a larger trial. Another common use of a pilot trial is to test two or three different blends to determine which is more efficacious and thus should undergo further testing.

Companies sometimes use pilots as a way of financing full trials. If the results are solid, companies can use them to secure additional funding to complete the full trial.

Generally speaking, pilot trials are useful to demonstrate how products will react for specific endpoints but lack the sample size required to achieve statistical significance. Depending on how the pilot is designed, these data may or may not be used in the full trial.

These are some of the reasons companies might begin with a pilot trial, then proceed to a full trial, which offers regulatory protection.

Product Testing

Product testing refers to a laboratory test of the blend or product. Companies are often interested in certifying the precise details of their blend in order to validate the blending procedure. Questions regarding the quality of the manufacturing process can be answered to some degree through a paper trail, but full verification requires the work of an experienced laboratory. Blends can be tested against the paper-trail documentation such as receipts, packing slips, and labels. This information lends support to a company's marketing claims and facilitates sound decision making regarding which raw ingredients to use in the future.

Laboratories are located throughout the country and can be found through referrals from industry consultants. Companies may require the advice of an experienced and perhaps independent research scientist to interpret the data. This depends upon the laboratory and how its reports are developed.

Open-Label Trials

An open-label trial is where both the subjects and staff know that the subjects are taking the actual product. In these cases, there is no placebo or control involved.

Open-label trials are used either in the pilot phase or in the case in which the biology of the product makes a control less of an issue. In the case of a product being assessed for enzymatic activity, one can employ an open-label approach by taking baseline levels, giving the product designed to change enzyme levels, then measuring after the desired duration has been achieved. A disadvantage of open-label trials is that they are considered less of a gold standard. The primary advantage is budgetary.

The Gold-Standard Design: Randomized, Placebo-Controlled, Blinded Clinical Trial

A gold-standard clinical trial is a pharmaceutical-level type trial employing a control group, IRB approval, randomization, blinding, oversight, and more. The name comes from the idea that all strategies that can improve validity and reliability are employed together. Embedded in this category is the type of study that can include parallel or crossover design features.

Randomized, placebo-controlled, blinded trials are those that typically decide if a new drug will make it into the marketplace and are generally reported in scientific literature. For a new drug, the FDA has defined four levels of required trials involving efficacy and safety and multi-site studies. Each may require months or years of planning, execution, and analysis. In addition, at any point throughout the process the drug may require changes in the following areas:

- dosing or delivery
- the identification or definition of contraindication
- changes in the endpoints
- changes in the laboratory values
- other parameters

This is an important contributing factor as to why only a fraction of all drugs make it through the FDA process and become licensed. There is obviously higher cost associated with the increase in scientific credibility. Costs can be in the millions of dollars.

All gold-standard trials include:

- randomization
- placebo control
- blinding
- physician oversight
- bi-weekly status reports

Discretionary options are:

- independent statistical analysis
- independent study oversight
- laboratory testing
- special medical testing
- resting metabolic rate
- body fat and lean muscle mass (as measured using Life Measurement, Inc.'s Bod Pod)
- computerized neurocognitive testing

Statistical Analysis

Careful and systematic analysis of study findings is essential to understand the nature of consumer benefit, to develop supportable claims, and to identify future problems. An individual with proper credentials and training in supplement research is required to conduct the review of research findings and isolate the important findings upon which one may rely.

Publishing Trial Results

Most important research results are published in some form to support the advancement of medical industry knowledge. This is research that other scientists rely on and that supplement companies use to determine which ingredients and blends to market. Publishing helps to promote public safety because results are available to other scientists and the general public. Knowing about poor results or adverse events from other studies can save money and prevent suffering. Finally, publishing results in reputable journals lends credibility to the results.

Research Funding

In some cases, state and federal funding is available to conduct follow-up research to confirm questionable findings or to study a new area identified through a completed study. Securing grant opportunities is a long-range strategy because this process may take several years to get off the ground, but the rewards are increased credibility and subsequent marketing opportunities.

Legal Action

Federal Trade Commission (FTC) law requires advertising claims to be supported by science. It is not sufficient to rely on existing data. If a product makes claims associated with sexual health, weight loss, or sleep quality, all considered health matters, then both the individual ingredients and the combined mixture of ingredients require substantiation. Existing medical conditions of study subjects can also be the cause for costly legal action. Experienced researchers know how to identify and control for these concerns. Review of past research prior to clinical testing and vigilance about the most common contra-indicated medical conditions during the trial prevents costly legal claims. Ethical considerations may require removing ingredients while in the production stage and/or the use of proper label warnings to protect consumers.

Lawsuits, regulatory fines, and lost consumer confidence are costly and can have long-lasting negative effects on a company's ability to continue sales or develop new products to keep up with new developments. Many companies learn this lesson the hard way.

Sources

- "Bias." Wikipedia. http://www.wikipedia.com (accessed July, 2007).
- Elston, R. C., and Johnson, W. D. *Essentials of Biostatistics*, 2nd edition. Philadelphia: F.A. Davis Company, 1994.
- "Epidemiology." Wikipedia. http://www.wikipedia.com (accessed July, 2007).
- Fairchild, A. L., and R. Bayer. "Uses and Abuses of Tuskegee." May 1999, Vol. 284. no. 5416, pp 919-921.

Science magazine. Accessed on sciencemag.com July 2007.

- Friis, R. H., and T. A. Sellers. *Epidemiology for Public Health Practice*. Boston: Jones and Bartlett Publishers, 2004.

- Gordis, L. *Epidemiology*, 2nd edition. Philadelphia: W.B. Saunders Company, 2000.

- Greenberg, Raymond S., et al. *Medical Epidemiology*. New York: Lange Medical Books/McGraw-Hill, 2001.

- Hulley, Stephen B., and Steven R Cummings. *Designing Clinical Research*. Baltimore: Williams and Wilkens, 1988.

- Lilienfeld, Abraham M. and David. *Foundations of Epidemiology*, 3rd edition. New York: Oxford University Press, 1988.

- Meinert, Curtis L. *Clinical Trials: Design, Conduct, and Analysis*. New York: Oxford University Press, 1986.

- "Scientific Method." Merriam Webster's Online Dictionary. http:// www.m-w.com/dictionary/scientific%20 method (accessed July, 2007).

- "Scientific Method." Wikipedia. http://www.wikipedia. com (accessed July, 2007).

- Sokal, Robert R., and F. James Rohlf. *Biometry*, 2nd edition. New York: W.H. Freeman and Company, 1980.

James M. Blum is an epidemiologist and principal consultant of DSRG with thirty-seven years of experience in both the medical field and dietary supplement research.

APPENDIX 2

FETAL PROGRAMMING: THE DEVELOPMENTAL ORIGINS OF ADULT DISEASE

Human beings, like other living creatures, are able to respond and acclimate to their environment. A good example of this is the way human metabolism gradually slows when fewer calories are consumed. A more extreme example is the case of Ralph Flores and Helen Klaben, the plane crash survivors who didn't eat for thirty days (which you read about in chapter 1). The ability to temporarily slow their metabolism and use stored fat allowed them to live through this ordeal. Being able to adapt metabolism to better cope with various environmental challenges is an illustration of human metabolic plasticity—an ability that is advantageous for survival.

This facility is also present in early life; in fact, it is even well developed in the womb—often with a special twist. Let me explain what I mean.

During pregnancy there are special times called "critical periods." If the fetus is exposed to environmental pressures during these critical stages of development in the womb, it can adapt. Unlike the temporary metabolic changes Flores and Klaben experienced, however, the metabolic alterations induced during these prenatal special windows of time remain *fixed*, which means they last forever. It is as if intrauterine stress gives the fetus a preliminary "snapshot" that portends what life will be like outside the womb. The fetus responds by adapting its metabolism to better cope with the life after birth it anticipates based on this snapshot. The existence of such critical periods of enhanced sensitivity in utero, associated with the ability to permanently reprogram physiologic responses, is designed to help the child better survive in a potentially hostile world.

The different size of newborn babies is a good example of developmental plasticity. The size of the mother constrains the growth of babies; otherwise, normal birth could not occur. Small women have small babies. But babies may also be small because they are not provided with adequate nutrients for growth. As R. A. McCance wrote long ago, "The size attained in utero depends on the services which the mother is able to supply. These are mainly food and accommodation." (See "Food, Growth and Time," *Lancet* 2 (1962): 621–26.) Since maternal height and pelvic dimensions are not usually predictors of the baby's long-term health, research into the developmental origins of adult disease has focused on the nutritional environment of the baby. Around the world, size at birth in relation to gestational age is a valid indicator of fetal nutrition.

The functional adaptations the fetus can exhibit include changes in the development of the various organs and bodily systems. For example, if the mother is poorly nourished during her pregnancy, she signals to her unborn child that the environment it is about to enter will likely be harsh and food might be scarce. The baby responds by making precise adaptive changes, such as reduced body size and altered metabolism, which will help it to survive food shortages after birth, because a smaller body and a slower metabolism can get by with fewer calories. This metabolic plasticity gives the species the ability to make short-term adaptations. However, as we will see, these same adaptations can be associated with adverse health consequences later in life.

Since the ability of the mother to nourish her baby is partially determined when she herself is in utero, the human fetus receives a "weather forecast" of future circumstances based not only on current conditions but also on conditions that existed a couple of decades earlier. So you can see how fetal programming effects can span several generations.

This body of information helps us to understand the basis for the developmental origins of some important adult diseases. The programming of adult fat accumulation is one such process. For example, a child born small is more likely to grow up small but with enhanced fat accumulation, especially in the abdominal region. Small babies are also at greater risk of developing high blood pressure and diabetes.

Numerous researchers have contributed to the fetal origins theory of disease causation. This theory proposes that the beginnings of certain adult diseases can be traced to the developmental responses induced by stresses during critical time windows in utero (or shortly after birth). The precise reasons for this are unclear.

One explanation suggests that under adverse gestational circumstances the allocation of scarce resources is directed preferentially to certain organs or processes, such as brain growth, at the expense of other organs. For example, if the brain is given priority, the kidneys may suffer. They might end up with fewer cells and fewer glomeruli—the functional units of the kidney. Over time this could lead to hyperfiltration of blood through each glomerulus, which injures the kidney. Alterations in the function of the kidney then contribute to hormonal changes that produce high blood pressure. In fact, these changes have been documented in animal models.

Another possible explanation by which slowed growth may produce later disease is via a resetting of the hormonal milieu in the fetus. Insulin resistance—a condition wherein the body responds less efficiently to the hormone insulin—is associated with low birth weight. One manifestation of insulin resistance is that glucose is not properly transported into muscle cells. As a result, it builds up to higher levels in the blood, which makes more glucose available for the fetal brain. Thus, insulin resistance in utero acts as a protective mechanism for the brain. However, later in life it may be associated with excess fat accumulation and other metabolic disorders such as heart disease, hypertension, and diabetes.

One example of how changes in fetal nutrition (as reflected by birth weight) affect health many years later is a study published in the *Journal of the American College of Nutrition*. It assessed the risk of developing diabetes in sixty-four-year-old men in relation to their birth weight. The smallest babies were 6.6 times more likely to become diabetic six decades later.

It should be noted that the development of certain diseases in adult life is not merely conditioned by the intrauterine environment; events during childhood and subsequent lifestyle choices made during adulthood also have an impact. It is even conceivable that being born small may make a person more sensitive to later metabolic influences such as stress, diet, or smoking.

Fetal *undernutrition* can have a dramatic impact on subsequent illness by permanently altering the body's physiology. It is also the case that fetal *overnutrition* can adversely impact future health. In most Western countries this is of greater concern today because bigger and fatter babies are much more common. A paper in the medical journal *Obstetrics and Gynecology* documented a 23 percent increase in large babies (related to fetal overnutrition) during a ten-year interval. This increase was associated with an 11 percent increase in maternal body mass index, or BMI, which is an indicator of maternal size.

With the rising prevalence of maternal obesity in most developed countries, more recent studies have been investigating the impact of overnutrition on the development of adult diseases. The results suggest that the offspring of obese mothers are more likely to become obese. They are also at increased risk for developing diabetes and what the medical community refers to as the metabolic syndrome: a constellation of disorders including obesity, diabetes, high blood pressure, elevated serum triglyceride levels, low HDL cholesterol levels, and small, dense LDL particles. The metabolic syndrome is likewise a potent risk factor for the development of cardiovascular disease. However, the reason for the transfer of risk from mother to child is currently not well understood.

Maternal diabetes, gestational diabetes (the development of diabetes during pregnancy), maternal obesity, and excessive maternal weight gain during pregnancy are important risk factors for having a large baby. All these conditions have in common either intermittent or sustained hyperglycemia (elevated blood sugar levels) in the mother. High glucose levels in the maternal circulation induce the transfer of increased amounts of glucose across the placenta (the link between the maternal and fetal circulation) into the fetus. This is equivalent to feeding the developing baby excessive amounts of sugar. As a result, there is a rise in fetal insulin levels.

It is important to mention at this juncture that insulin is the primary growth hormone in the fetus. Hence, high insulin levels drive body growth during pregnancy. In addition, as has already been seen, insulin is the fat-storage hormone. High insulin levels enhance the storage of fat in babies as well as adults.

Ultrasound (US) is a noninvasive form of imaging that can take pictures of small babies in utero without causing any harm. The technology has improved to the point where US images can be used to determine the fat mass of the developing infant. Investigators evaluated fat mass in neonates born to mothers with diabetes and in those who developed diabetes during the pregnancy (gestational diabetes). They determined that higher blood glucose in the mother during pregnancy is associated with fatter babies. What is particularly disturbing is that, *even when their birth weight is normal*, these infants have a higher fat mass compared to babies born to mothers without elevated glucose.

Another study compared fetal body fat in nondiabetic mothers manifesting only *slightly abnormal* glucose levels with that in mothers with *normal* blood glucose levels. They found elevated body fat in the babies of the mothers with only slightly elevated blood glucose levels. As noted in the *American Journal of Obstetrics and Gynecology*, this increase in body fat may be a significant risk for obesity in early childhood and possibly in later life. Thus, in addition to maternal body mass, the expectant mother's blood glucose levels are a major determinant of fetal fat mass. It appears that the associated rise in fetal insulin levels is contributing to fat babies in the same manner it produces fat adults.

In addition to programming babies to become very efficient at storing fat, fetal overnutrition can produce other physiologic alterations. It has been proposed that exposure of the fetus to an excessive nutrient supply during critical windows of development may result in permanent changes within the appetite regulatory system in the brain of the newborn baby. This has been investigated in animal models, which have demonstrated changes in the expression of neuropeptides that regulate food intake. This represents another mechanism whereby fetal overnutrition may lead to a subsequent increase in childhood and adult obesity.

A recent paper published in the *Journal of Physiology* described another animal study that is germane to the current discussion. When rats were fed a "junk food" diet during pregnancy and lactation, their offspring were born fat and had elevated levels of glucose, insulin, and cholesterol. It is important to note that the mother rats in this study were not diabetic. They were normal mother rats that were exposed to a diet that produced high blood sugar and insulin levels. This is the type of diet many human mothers consume—often with the same results.

With these insights, what can be done to help curb the

obesity epidemic we are experiencing? It is evident that processes that predispose newborn babies to become overweight and develop diabetes and high blood pressure as adults originate before birth. This important observation should not be ignored! Women who intend to become pregnant should strive to be of normal weight and should avoid gaining excessive weight during pregnancy. They should consider following a program of regular exercise, under the direction of a doctor, throughout the pregnancy. If this recommendation is followed, the offspring of these women will have lower fat mass than the offspring born to women who do not exercise.

Women who intend to bear children should also eat a diet that maintains normal blood glucose and insulin levels. Since the Feed Your Brain Lose Your Belly diet is designed to control glucose and insulin levels, it is a reasonable diet to consider during pregnancy. However, because of the potent metabolic effects it can produce, in this context it should only be followed under the supervision of a physician.

If these prescriptions are taken seriously, we will be giving the next generation its best opportunity to lead a happy and healthy life.

APPENDIX 3

SUGGESTED READING

Baker, L.D., D.J. Cross, S. Minoshima, D. Belongia, G.S. Watson, and S. Craft. "Insulin Resistance and Alzheimer-like Reductions in Regional Cerebral Glucose Metabolism for Cognitively Normal Adults With Prediabetes or Early Type 2 Diabetes." Arch Neurol (2010) Sep 13 [Epub ahead of print].

Berry, M. N., D. G. Clark, A. R. Grivell, and P. G. Wallace. "The Contribution of Hepatic Metabolism to Diet-Induced Thermogenesis." Metabolism 34 (1985): 141–147.

Biessels, G. J., B. Bravenboer, and W. H. Gispen. "Glucose, Insulin and the Brain: Modulation of Cognition and Synaptic Plasticity in Health and Disease: A Preface." European Journal of Pharmacology 490 (2004): 1–4.

Boden, G., K. Sargrad, C. Homko, M. Mozzoli, and T. P. Stein. "Effect of a Low-Carbohydrate Diet on Appetite, Blood Glucose Levels, and Insulin Resistance in Obese Patients with Type 2 Diabetes." Ann Int Med 142 (2005): 403–411.

Byrnes, Stephen. "Are Saturated Fats Really Dangerous for You?" http://www.mercola.com/2002/feb/23/vegetarianism_myths_06.htm

Cahill, G. F. Jr, and R. L. Veech. "Ketoacids? Good Medicine?" Trans Am Clin Climatol Assoc 114 (2003): 149–161.

Carro, E., and I. Torres-Aleman. "The Role of Insulin and Insulin–like Growth Factor 1 in the Molecular and Cellular Mechanisms Underlying the Pathology of Alzheimer's Disease." European Journal of Pharmacology 490 (2004): 127–133.

Convit, A., O. T. Wolf, C. Tarshish, and M. J. de Leon. "Reduced Glucose Tolerance is Associated with Poor Memory Performance and Hippocampal Atrophy Among Normal Elderly." Proceedings of the National Academy of Sciences of the United States of America 100 (2003): 2019–2022.

Craft, S. "Insulin Resistance and Cognitive Impairment." Archives of Neurology 62 (2005): 1043–1044.

———"Insulin Resistance Syndrome and Alzheimer's Disease: Age-and Obesity-Related Effects on Memory, Amyloid and Inflammation." Neurobiology of Aging 26S (2005): S65–S69.

Craft, S., and G. S. Watson. "Insulin and Neurodegenerative Disease: Shared and Specific Mechanisms." Lancet 3 (2004): 169–178.

Cunnane, S. C. "Metabolic and Health Implications of Moderate Ketosis and the Ketogenic Diet." Prostaglandins, Leukotrienes and Essential Fatty Acids 70 (2004): 233–234.

———"Metabolism of Polyunsaturated Fatty Acids and Ketogenesis: An Emerging Connection." Prostaglandins, Leukotrienes and Essential Fatty Acids 70 (2004): 237–241.

———"New Developments in Alpha-Linolenate Metabolism with Emphasis on the Importance of Beta-Oxidation and Carbon Recycling." World Rev Nutr Diet 88 (2001): 178–183.

———"Problems with Essential Fatty Acids: Time for a New Paradigm?" Prog Lipid Res 42 (2003): 544–568.

de Rooij, S.R., H. Wouters, J.E. Yonker, R.C. Painter, and T.J. Roseboom. "Prenatal Undernutrition and Cognitive Function in Late Adulthood." Proceedings of the National Academy of Sciences USA 107 (2010): 16757-16758.

Enig, Mary. Know Your Fats: The Complete Primer for Understanding the Nutrition of Fats, Oils and Cholesterol. Bethesda: Bethesda Press, 2000.

Fishel, M. A., G. S. Watson, T. J. Montine, Q. Wang, P. S. Green, J. J. Kulstad, D. G. Cook, E. R. Peskind, L. D. Baker, D. Goldgaber, W. Nie, S. Asthana, S. R. Plymate, and S. Craft. "Hyperinsulinemia Promotes Synchronous Increases in Central Inflammation and Beta-Amyloid in Normal Adults." Archives of Neurology 62 (2005): 1539–1544.

Freemantle, E., M. Vandal, J Tremblay-Mercier, S. Tremblay, J. C. Blachere, M. E. Begin, J. T. Brenna, A. Windust, and S. C. Cunnane. "Omega-3 Fatty Acids, Energy Substrates and Brain Function During Aging." Prostaglandins, Leukotrienes and Essential Fatty Acids 75 (2006): 213–220.

Gardner, C. D., A. Kiazand, S. Alhassan, S. Kim, R. S. Stafford, R. R. Balise, H. C. Kraemer, and A. C. King. "Comparison of the Atkins, Zone, Ornish, and LEARN Diets for Change in Weight and Related Risk Factors Among Overweight Premenopausal Women." JAMA 297 (2007): 969–977.

Geroldi, C., G. B. Frisoni, G. Paolisso, S. Bandinelli, J. M. Guralnik, and L. Ferrucci. "Insulin Resistance in Cognitive Impairment." Archives of Neurology 62 (2005): 1067–1072.

Haist, R. E., and C. H. Best. "Carbohydrate Metabolism and Insulin." In The Physiological Basis of Medical Practice, 8th edition. (pp. 1329–1367). Edited by C. H. Best and N. M. Taylor. Baltimore: Williams and Wilkins, 1996.

Han, J. R., B. Deng, J. Sun, C. G. Chen, B. E. Corkey, J. L. Kirkland, J. Ma, and W. Guo. "Effects of Dietary Medium-Chain Triglyceride on Weight Loss and Insulin Sensitivity in a Group of Moderately Overweight Free-Living Type 2 Diabetic Chinese Subjects." Metabolism 56 (2007): 985–991.

Hanssen, P. "Treatment of Obesity by a Diet Relatively Poor in Carbohydrates." Acta Medica Scandinavica 88 (1936): 97–106.

Henderson, S. T. "High Carbohydrate Diets and Alzheimer's Disease." Medical Hypotheses 62 (2004): 689–700.

Kahn, B. B., and J. Flier. "Obesity and Insulin Resistance." J Clin Invest 106 (2000): 473–481.

Kasai, M., H. Maki, N. Nosaka, T. Aoyama, K. Ooyama, H. Uto, M. Okazaki, O. Igarashi, and K. Kondo. "Effect of Medium-Chain Triglycerides on the Postprandial Triglyceride Concentration in Healthy Men." Biosci Biotechnol Biochem 67 (2003): 46–53.

Keys, A., J. Brozek, A. Henschel, O. Mickelsen, and H. L. Taylor. The Biology of Human Starvation. 2 vols. Minneapolis: University of Minnesota Press, 1950.

McCall, A. L. "Altered Glycemia and Brain-Uptake and Potential Relevance to the Aging Brain." Neurobiology of Aging 26S (2005): S70–S75.

McGarry, J. D., and D. W. Foster. "Regulation of Hepatic Fatty Acid Oxidation and Ketone Body Production." Annu Rev Biochem 49 (1980): 395–420.

Mokdad, A. H., B. A. Bowman, E. S. Ford, F. Vinicor, J. S. Marks, and J. P. Koplan. "The Continuing Epidemic of Obesity in the United States." JAMA 284 (2000): 1650–1651.

Mokdad, A. H., M. K. Serdula, W. H. Dietz, B. A. Bowman, J. S. Marks, and J. P. Koplan. "The Spread of the Obesity Epidemic in the United States, 1991–1998." JAMA 282 (1999): 1519–1522.

Morris, M. C., D. A. Evans, J. L. Bienias, C. C. Tangney, D. A. Bennett, R. S. Wilson, N. Aggarwal, and J. Schneider. "Consumption of Fish and N-3 Fatty Acids and Risk of Incident Alzheimer Disease." Archives of Neurology 60 (2003): 940–946.

Morris, M. C., D. A. Evans, C. C. Tangney, J. L. Bienias, and R. S. Wilson. "Fish Consumption and Cognitive Decline with Age in a Large Community Study." Archives of Neurology 62 (2005): 1849–1853.

Reaven, G. A. "Banting Lecture1988: Role of Insulin Resistance in Human Disease." Diabetes 37 (1988): 1595–1607.

Reaven, G. M. "The Insulin Resistance Syndrome: Definition and Dietary Approaches to Treatment." Annual Review of Nutrition 25 (2005): 391–406.

Reger, M. A., S. T. Henderson, C. Hale, B. Cholerton, L. D. Baker, G. S. Watson, K. Hyde, D. Chapman, and S. Craft. "Effects of Beta-Hydroxybutyrate on Cognition in Memory-Impaired Adults." Neurobiology of Aging 25 (2004): 311–314.

Reger, M. A., G. S. Watson, W. H. Frey, L. D. Baker, B. Cholerton, M. L. Keeling, D. A. Belongia, M. A. Fishel, S. R. Plymate, G. D. Schellenberg, M. M. Cherrier, and S. Craft. "Effects of Intranasal Insulin on Cognition in Memory-Impaired Older Adults: Modulation by APOE Genotype." Neurobiology of Aging 27 (2006): 451–458.

Ruderman, N., D. Chisholm, X. Pi-Sunyer, and S. Schneider. "The Metabolically–Obese, Normal-Weight Individual Revisited." Diabetes 47 (1998): 699–713.

Ruderman, N. B., S. H. Schneider, and P. Berchtold. "The Metabolically-Obese, Normal-Weight Individual." Am J Clin Nutr 34 (1981): 1617–1622.

Scharrer, E. "Control of Food Intake by Fatty Acid Oxidation and Ketogenesis." Nutrition 15 (1999): 704–714.

Shishodia, S., G. Sethi, and B. A. Aggarwal. "Curcumin: Getting Back to the Roots." Annals of the New York Academy of Science 1056 (2005): 206–217.

St-Onge, M. P., and A. Bosarge. "Weight-Loss Diet that Includes Consumption of Medium-Chain Triacylglycerol Oil Leads to a Greater Rate of Weight and Fat Loss than Does Olive Oil." Am J Clin Nutr 87 (2008): 621–626.

St-Onge, M. P., A. Bosarge, L. L. Goree, and B. Darnell. "Medium Chain Triglyceride Oil Consumption as Part of a Weight Loss Diet Does Not Lead to an Adverse Metabolic Profile When Compared With Olive Oil." J Am Coll Nutr 27 (2008): 547-552.

St-Onge, M. P., R. Ross, W. D. Parsons, and P. J. Jones. "Medium-Chain Triglycerides Increase Energy Expenditure and Decrease Adiposity in Overweight Men." Obes Res 11 (2003): 395-402.

Taubes, Gary. Good Calories, Bad Calories: Challenging the Conventional Wisdom on Diet, Weight Control, and Disease. New York: Knopf, 2007.

Yehuda, S. "Omega-6/Omega-3 Ratio and Brain-Related Functions." World Review of Nutrition and Dietetics 92 (2003): 37–56.

Yehuda, S., S. Rabinovitz, and D. I. Mostofsky. "Essential Fatty Acids and the Brain: From Infancy to Aging." Neurobiology of Aging 26, suppl. 1 (2005): 98–102.

Veech, R. L. "The Therapeutic Implications of Ketone Bodies: The Effects of Ketone Bodies in Pathological Conditions: Ketogenic Diet, Redox States, Insulin Resistance and Mitochondrial Metabolism." Prostaglandins, Leukotrienes and Essential Fatty Acids 70 (2004): 309–319.

Veech, R. L., B. Chance, Y. Kashiwaya, H. A. Lardy, and G. F. Cahill Jr. "Ketone Bodies, Potential Therapeutic Uses." IUBMB Life 51 (2001): 241–247.

INDEX

ABOUT THE AUTHOR

Larry McCleary, MD, was acting chief of pediatric neurosurgery at Denver Children's Hospital. After graduating from Dartmouth College, he performed postgraduate work in theoretical physics at Boston University. He went to medical school at the State University of New York–Buffalo, did his surgical internship at the University of Minnesota, and completed his residency in neurosurgery at New York University/Bellevue Hospital Center.

Dr. McCleary's other books include *The Brain Trust Program: A Scientifically Based Three-Part Plan to Improve Memory, Elevate Mood, Enhance Attention, Alleviate Migraine & Menopausal Symptoms and Boost Mental Energy* (Perigee Press, 2007) and the two-volume set *Bald Is Beautiful: The Shining Stars Foundation Guide for Living with Childhood Cancer* (2009), which can be ordered online at www.ShiningStarsFoundation.org. He has also published numerous medical articles in *Cancer*, the *Journal of Neurosurgery*, *Neurosurgery*, *Neurology*, and the *American Journal of Neuroradiology*, among other periodicals.

Dr. McCleary holds several patents for nutritional supplements and is the medical director for the Shining Stars Foundation, a nonprofit organization located in Colorado that provides programs for children with cancer and other life-threatening diseases.